Feeling Good
about the Way You Look

Feeling Good about the Way You Look

A Program for Overcoming Body Image Problems

Sabine Wilhelm, PhD

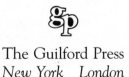

The Guilford Press
New York   London

© 2006 Sabine Wilhelm
Published by The Guilford Press
A Division of Guilford Publications, Inc.
72 Spring Street, New York, NY 10012
www.guilford.com

Library of Congress Cataloging-in-Publication Data

Wilhelm, Sabine.
    Feeling good about the way you look : a program for overcoming body image
problems / Sabine Wilhelm.
        p.   cm.
    Includes index.
    ISBN-10: 1-59385-294-0   ISBN-13: 978-1-59385-294-8 (trade cloth)
    ISBN-10: 1-57230-730-7   ISBN-13: 978-1-57230-730-8 (trade paper)
    1. Body image.   I. Title.
    BF697.5.B63W54 2006
    646.7—dc22   2005036320

For Arun, Sarah, and Marc

Contents

Preface

I wrote this book for people who feel they worry too much about how they look and want to do something about it. If concerns about your appearance have a negative effect on your self-esteem, or get in the way of your enjoying life, this book can help. You should also consider reading this book if your dissatisfaction with your appearance leads you to avoid certain social activities, or if you're spending excessive amounts of time or money on beauty products or strategies to improve your appearance, from hair removal to muscle building.

Some people are only mildly dissatisfied with their appearance; for others, concerns about their appearance can be completely incapacitating. Regardless of where you fall along a continuum between these extremes, the strategies described in this book can help you. I've used them with people whose concerns aren't too severe and with those diagnosed with body dysmorphic disorder (BDD, a severely distressing preoccupation with certain aspects of one's appearance).

You may have picked up this book because you have a relative or friend with body image concerns, and you're worried about how the problem is affecting him or her. This book will help you understand the problem enough to determine whether and how you can help. Chapter 11 is just for you, but all the preceding chapters will be informative too. You may want to recommend the program in this book to your relative or friend after reading through it, especially if you believe you can support your family member or friend in overcoming dissatisfaction and distress. If the person you're concerned about is not sure about trying a self-help program, the Resources section at the back of the book can help both of you locate a qualified therapist. Therapists who don't have a lot of experience with body image concerns, in fact, may find this book a useful guide too.

Feeling Good about the Way You Look differs from other books about body image in a number of ways. Many of the other books available focus primarily on concerns related to weight and body shape and are geared predominantly toward women. This book focuses on appearance concerns in a much broader sense. It doesn't matter whether you are male or female, or whether you are ashamed of your skin, hair, lips, or any other body part. This book can provide you with a new understanding of your problem. But it also offers concrete strategies for overcoming your distress in the form of a step-by-step self-help program. To develop the program laid out in this book, I've integrated what I learned from the body image literature, from my own research studies, and from my patients. In 1998, I founded the BDD Clinic and Research Unit at Massachusetts General Hospital/Harvard Medical School in Boston. Since then, I have evaluated or treated over 300 patients with BDD or related disorders. I have also conducted several studies on the treatment of BDD and related problems. My research focuses on the nature of BDD and, in particular, on how people with BDD think and process information. The large majority of the patients treated in our BDD program experience a substantial decrease in their appearance dissatisfaction. They also learn to control excessive appearance rituals and reduce their avoidance behaviors. In this book you'll find versions of my clinical strategies modified for self-help. Depending on the severity of your dissatisfaction with your appearance, you may be able to use this book alone or as an adjunct to regular visits with a clinician. If you are not already seeing a therapist about your appearance concerns, and you have any doubt about your ability or willingness to try self-help, please find a qualified therapist with experience in treating body image concerns like BDD; you'll find guidance on locating such a therapist at the back of this book.

The journey toward overcoming your appearance obsessions and related distress may be challenging at times. But hang in there. It may take hard work, but if you persevere, you can remove worry about how you look from the center of your life and free yourself to enjoy the days ahead.

Acknowledgments

This book would not have been written without the help of many individuals and organizations. First of all, I want to thank all my patients who have shared their personal stories, deepest secrets, and triumphs over the years. They have taught me most of what I know about this problem. I will always be impressed by their strength, courage, and determination to succeed.

I am very pleased to have The Guilford Press as my publisher and feel indebted to Kitty Moore for seeing the value of a self-help book on body image concerns and for her guidance throughout the project. Christine Benton's thoughtful editing and outstanding suggestions and queries have made this book so much better than it would otherwise have been.

Many thanks to Dr. Michael Otto for encouraging me to write this book, for recommending me to The Guilford Press, and for providing helpful suggestions on Chapters 1 and 6.

I would also like to recognize Dr. Katharine A. Phillips for all the important research she has done on BDD, for being such a great collaborator, and for editing Chapter 10 on pharmacotherapy. Special thanks also to my teacher, research collaborator, and friend, Gail Steketee, for everything she has taught me about cognitive-behavioral therapy research and for her guidance over the years.

I am grateful to my talented coworkers at Massachusetts General Hospital for their support and enthusiasm for my work on BDD. Special thanks to my mentor, Dr. Michael Jenike, for his encouragement over the years and for his contribution to Chapter 10 on pharmacotherapy. I thank the chief of psychiatry at Massachusetts General Hospital, Dr. Jerrold Rosenbaum, for his support and for providing me with the space for my research activities. Thank you to Dr. Ulrike Buhlmann and Dr. Jeanne Fama for all their hard work. Many thanks also to Kara Watts and Elana Golan for reading portions of an earlier draft of this book. I also want to thank the National Institute of Mental Health and Massachusetts General Hospital for supporting my research.

Finally, this book would not exist without the encouragement of my wonderful family. First, I want to thank my husband, Arun Hiranandani, for his patience and support on the many nights and weekends I spent writing this book. I also wish to thank my children, Sarah and Marc, for being there and for sharing me with my work. Many thanks to my parents, Richard and Paula Wilhelm, who have always encouraged me to take on new challenges.

Chapter 1

For the Sake
of Appearance

Emily*, a beautiful 23-year-old medical student, is preoccupied with her skin. She does fine talking to others when she thinks her skin is clear. But when she has a pimple, even speaking to friends makes her nervous—she's sure they're staring at her face. "Why can't my skin look like hers?" she asks herself constantly. "Why can't it be smooth?" Unfortunately, looking at others usually doesn't help, because they seem to look so much better, and this just reinforces her feelings of defectiveness. Emily spends a lot of time checking her appearance in mirrors, and what she sees determines how she feels. Whenever she discovers a new imperfection on her skin, she feels anxious and disappointed, and thinks she looks "repulsive." Blemishes are "really disgusting" to her, and she tries to remove them by picking at her skin. Sometimes the picking itself causes skin irritations, which she then covers up with makeup. She feels particularly bad about some scars she caused during a recent picking episode, because now she's "responsible for making the problem even worse." She blames herself and now thinks even more about her imperfections. "I have these deep holes in my skin. This looks so abnormal. Really disfigured. Everyone will think: Look what she did to her face! What a freak!"

When Emily feels really bad about the scars or a pimple, she keeps asking her boyfriend, "Can you see it? How bad is it?" He usually tells her he can't see anything and she looks great, but lately he's been getting fed up with having to answer the same questions over and over. Emily doesn't believe him anyway: "He's just trying to be nice," she explains. He's also getting tired of missing out

*All patient names and identifying characteristics have been changed.

on social events because Emily won't leave the house if she feels her appearance isn't perfect. Now she's afraid he might break up with her if all this keeps up, but she doesn't know how to stop worrying so much about the way she looks.

Peter is a smart young lawyer with an attractive smile. He's a high achiever and well liked by his colleagues, who sometimes wonder why he always attends movies and parties alone—when he shows up at all. Peter claims that he has too much work to socialize. The truth is, he's afraid to meet new people. He hates his hair and is thoroughly convinced that no one could ever be attracted to him because of his receding hairline. So he avoids asking women for dates, going out only when someone pursues him, then wondering why anyone *would* pursue him: "What's wrong with her? Does she feel sorry for me?" Once he's on a date, he can't concentrate enough to converse, because all he can think is "She's staring at my hair . . . I'm the only one here who's balding . . . I wish I were invisible." Needless to say, second dates are few and far between.

Now Peter's obsession with his hair is starting to affect his job. Trying Rogaine and joining a hair club only left him glancing furtively into every reflective surface to check on the effects of the Rogaine. He inspects his hair from different angles and under different light, and sometimes even counts his hairs, which gets him stuck in front of the mirror for so long before work that he's often late. Recently he's started missing appointments with colleagues because he got mired in counting his hair in the office bathroom mirror. It bothers him that he's so obsessed with his hair, but he just can't stop thinking about it.

For Katie, a 40-year-old mother of three, her nose is the problem. She's already had two nose jobs and is considering a third. If only her nose were fixed correctly, she tells herself, her life would be OK: "I just can't tolerate being so ugly. I'd give anything to look pretty." Everyone else thought each nose shape she's had has looked fine. But after each surgery, Katie has gotten more preoccupied with her nose. Now she feels that her nose "looks really unnatural" and the surgeons "only made the problem worse and really screwed up my life." Over the years, her husband has tried reassurance, anger, pleas, and stony silence to change Katie's belief that her nose is repulsive—all to no avail. She worked as a nurse until about 5 years ago, but after the first nose surgery, she got so upset by her appearance that she couldn't go to work anymore. "My family is really hurting for the extra income, but I've declined many requests from my previous boss to come back. I just don't want my colleagues to see how I look now. I looked bad before the first surgery, but now I'm really repulsive."

At the gym, Ahmed is known as a serious weight-lifter who knows the correct protein supplement to take and the optimal strategy to develop one's "abs." He works out for hours with a detached seriousness that leaves him lonely in the gym despite his being a "regular." His workouts have swelled his chest and arms to the point that his dress shirts fit poorly, but what he sees in the mirror is "puny," "scrawny," "weak," or "unmanly." "Initially, the exercise was just meant to be a healthy thing, to stay in shape, you know?" he says. "But over time it got out of control. I needed to do more and more repetitions to get the feeling that I had completed a workout. I felt like I needed to spend every free minute working out. It sounds crazy, but lifting destroyed my marriage. I really loved my wife, and I still do, but after the lifting took over I never had time for her. I was always in the gym! You see, about 90% of my life revolves around my looks and my exercise. I'd much rather go to the gym than to a romantic dinner. If I ever had to miss a workout because I had to leave town or something, I got really depressed! So I simply would avoid anything that kept me away from the gym. . . . She didn't understand why we could never go out, never travel, and why I'd rather be at the gym than with her. So finally she divorced me! On top of that, I recently injured my knees from overtraining. I knew I had a problem because I just could not stop working out, even though the pain got really bad. Now it's so bad that I need surgery!"

As anyone who knows Emily, Peter, Katie, or Ahmed could tell you, they aren't crazy. They want the same things most of us want: to be happy, to have meaningful relationships, and to be productive members of society. But they are all struggling with a disturbed body image, and their lives are suffering as a direct consequence. Their body image problems are destroying their social relationships, their health, and their careers. Peter avoids dating and social activities, which isolates him increasingly, and now he's losing the goodwill of friends and colleagues, who are tired of his showing up late or canceling at the last minute because he's stuck in front of the mirror. Emily fears that her boyfriend will break up with her, and Ahmed's wife has already left him. Katie doesn't work even though the financial need is clear, and she can't tolerate being looked at by others.

They all know that something in their lives isn't as it should be. "Recently I got stuck in the office bathroom," says Peter, "and one of my coworkers saw me go in and not come out until 1 hour later! I was so embarrassed! I told him I had a stomach bug. But I'm tired of making excuses. I need to find another way to deal with this." Emily agrees, saying that she really doesn't want to lose her boyfriend but doesn't know how to stop obsessing and asking him for reassurance: "It feels out of my control." Ahmed knows that his appearance obsessions are responsible for his divorce and knee injury: "I've already messed up my health and my marriage because of being so worried about how I look. I need to do something about this now, because if I don't, I'll just keep lifting and ruin my knees again right after this surgery. I also want to date again at some point. But right now I'm way too shy to ask anyone out—and I can't imagine that any woman would tolerate my behavior!" Katie tells me, "I know I'm smart and I used to do a great job at work, but now I just sit at home and think about how ugly I am and how to fix my nose. I don't bring in any money, and believe me, we really need it! I feel like I let my family down. . . . I'd also be a much better wife and mother if I didn't always think about my nose. It's hard to focus on your family when your mind is always racing with thoughts about your looks. I am sick and tired of this! I want my life back!"

While these four are very aware that something is wrong in their lives, they don't know what to do about it. They can't free themselves from the hurtful perception that they are deformed, ugly, or repulsive. However, there's a difference between their perception (that is, their body image) and reality (their actual appearance), and the gap between that perception and reality is where the problem lies.

Your Word against Theirs: Body Image versus Appearance

Your body image is an inner view of your outer physical body. It's the perception you have of your own body, the way it appears to you. Your actual appearance has little relation to your sense of attractiveness. Being handsome or beautiful doesn't guarantee a good body image, and being homely doesn't automatically lead to a bad one. You can meet high standards of attractiveness without a flaw and still be dissatisfied with your looks, like the models I've worked with who were beautiful but still excessively concerned with some aspect of their appearance. Antonio, who works as a model, has told me, "I'm obsessed with my hair, in particular the sideburns. I want them to look stylish, so they have to be exactly symmetrical, not too long and not too short. Also, I can't have any thin spots. But if parts of my sideburns are too thick, it bothers me. I always give my stylist detailed instructions about how I want her to shape them. She probably thinks I'm nuts, because it takes forever until I'm satisfied with her work. But often she doesn't get it just right, and I then have to spend hours fixing them at home. I cut them and tweeze them. Usually I mess them up even further in this process and need to color in the parts that I don't like with an eyebrow pencil. I'm very ashamed of this! Nobody has ever said anything negative about my appearance, and I often get compliments about my looks. But still, if I think my sideburns are imperfect, it's difficult for me to leave the house. I guess I'm just terrified that anyone could notice that they aren't shaped correctly. I rarely miss work, but I'm trying to hold my head in a certain way to hide the bad spots if at all possible. I've disappointed my family so many times because I couldn't come to birthday parties or weddings because my sideburns weren't perfect."

You can be told repeatedly that you're good looking, yet you see an entirely different picture in the mirror. Why don't you see what others see when they look at you? Body image has only to do with how you see yourself, and people with a poor body image tend to focus only on the body parts they dislike, and disregard the ones they like or find acceptable. As a result, they get a very distorted view of themselves. One man once told me, "When I look in the mirror, my nose is all I can see. I feel like I'm nothing but a huge nose." Jorge, a successful, 38-year-old business owner, is certain that his skin is too red. He's very careful not to sit under bright lights and often applies cover-up. He is so preoccupied by worry about his skin tone, in fact, that he never pays attention to his nice build or attractive smile, features that everyone else sees immediately.

If Jorge's best friend told him to stop harping on his red skin and start noticing how many single women react so positively to his smile, his muscles, his great personality, and his impressive job, Jorge would say that it's only natural to notice your own flaws and do what you can to correct or hide them. It would be hard to argue with that response. What Jorge wouldn't admit, however, is that his skin can't really be flawed if no one else sees it that way. And even if it were flawed, should his dissatisfaction with it rule—and ruin—his life?

Your body image will affect how you think, feel, and act in certain situations. Jorge always notices men with paler skin and wishes he could look like them. Around others with "perfect" skin he feels inadequate and frustrated. If you have a good body image, you may be more self-confident, your self-esteem may be higher, and you might just like yourself better overall. If your body image is negative, you'll feel dissatisfied and preoccupied with your looks. You are likely to be self-critical and mentally beat yourself up for your flaws. You may monitor your environment closely for cues that relate to your appearance and may be very sensitive when anybody comments on it. You are likely to be insecure or anxious in certain social situations, and there are probably some things that you just avoid because they make you feel too uncomfortable. You may not feel as masculine or feminine as you wish, which may reduce sexual pleasure. You may feel that you are less acceptable as a person, or you may even feel discouraged about your future. On days when you think you look particularly bad, you may even have a hard time leaving the safety of your own home. You may compare yourself with people you consider more attractive, and spend a lot of time and effort trying to improve your looks. These patterns of thinking, feeling, and behaving will inevitably result in a sense of failure or inferiority. The more extreme your dissatisfaction and distress over your looks, and the longer you go on feeling this way, the more your life is likely to suffer as a result.

You're Not Alone

Hardly anyone goes through life completely satisfied with his or her appearance at all times. Dissatisfaction with appearance tends to arise at certain stages of life, such as puberty and middle age, and some people seem to fuss with their hair, skin, or clothing pretty much all the time, as a way of life. But chronic dissatisfaction or concern with appearance is a different matter, and it's alarmingly common.

Recently, Dr. Thomas Cash averaged body image questionnaire scores of students who participated in a variety of his research studies from 1996 to 2001. He found that 29% of nonblack women, 16% of nonblack men, and 17% of black women are dissatisfied with their looks. The sizable percentages of women and men who struggle with body dissatisfaction are likely related to the unrealistic body ideal being promoted by the media. We live in an image-conscious society that glorifies physical perfection. TV, radio, and magazines remind us daily to ensure that our breath is fresh, our hair is well styled, our stomachs are flat, and our blemishes are hidden. In a culture where bad hair can ruin a good day, body image distortions seem an almost natural, but tragic, outgrowth of constant attention to appearance. These body image distortions are an extreme magnification of normal concerns about appearance and cause a lot of suffering. What causes them is, of course, a lot more complicated than this brief recitation indicates, as discussed more fully in Chapter 2.

What's Normal and What's Not?

I've been working with individuals with body image disturbances since 1995. As a psychologist, naturally I see more people whose appearance concerns are severe than mild. But many people with body image concerns have relatively mild disturbances and lead relatively normal lives. Usually people with milder degrees of body image dissatisfaction don't consider their problem severe enough to initiate psychiatric treatment, but they still suffer. They think they have an embarrassing secret that no one can ever understand. They often fear that others might think of them as vain. And if they ever muster up the courage to disclose their secret, and others cannot see their flaws, they feel even more isolated. They may be our friends, our neighbors, or even family members.

If you have body image concerns, you're better off trying to set aside concerns about normality for now and instead examine how these concerns are impacting your own life. Discontentment with appearance extends from none or mild to moderate or severe. Thoughts about looks can occur several times per week and may happen many hours per day. Rituals performed in the name of beauty can range from eyebrow plucks to plastic surgeries. Checking the mirror can take several minutes to several hours per day. Some people spend a few dollars per month on cosmetics or hair replacement products; others spend several hundred dollars. Some individuals try to exercise occasionally, because they consider it healthy to train their heart and build their muscles. Others spend several hours per day in the gym and abuse steroids. For you, the important factor should be how much your preoccupation with your appearance is affecting your life. The difference between severe body image disturbance and other appearance concerns is merely a matter of degree, and the borders between normal and not can be blurry, especially in a society where most people are dissatisfied with some aspect of their appearance. It's sometimes difficult to decide whether distress and impairment as a result of appearance worries are still to be considered ordinary or should be classified as a psychiatric illness.

Jennifer has the soft features and tranquil dark eyes that we can easily imagine seeing in the pages of a fashion magazine. Her hair is brushed toward her face, and when speaking, she inclines her face downward, which gives her a look of seriousness, as if she's about to share a great confidence. This habit appears almost coquettish, a habit perhaps to draw attention. But attention from others is not only unwanted but also feared by Jennifer. She's hiding. She's hiding behind her carefully brushed hair, her perfectly applied makeup, and her carefully rehearsed tilt of the head. She's hiding in her house when she turns down invitations from friends. She's hiding her perceived ugliness, a feeling of ugliness that now centers on the color of her skin. She's convinced that her skin's too pale, and that she looks sick and tired. Jennifer is also extremely concerned with a scar on her left cheek. Although her friends and family are unable to see these defects, and honestly proclaim her attractiveness, these perceived flaws control Jennifer's life.

Jennifer used to work as an administrative assistant. Her boss mostly asked her to do paperwork and answer the phone, which she liked because she could work by herself. This way nobody could see her. Although Jennifer enjoyed her job, she was late almost every day because she got stuck in front of the mirror before leaving the house. In the morning, it often took her over 2 hours to put on her makeup. But she was convinced that she needed camouflaging to hide her perceived defects from others. Eventually Jennifer ended up getting fired. She tried out a few other jobs but ultimately left or got fired from each one.

Thereafter, things got even worse. Because she wasn't working any longer, she felt there was no reason to get up in the morning and spent half the day at home in bed. Her self-esteem plummeted, and her appearance concerns worsened. This only made her withdraw further. She started avoiding supermarkets and family events because she was so concerned about her appearance. She felt useless because she didn't work and got more and more embarrassed about the way she looked. As a result, she became really depressed.

Jennifer's body image disturbance is severe. Jennifer has body dysmorphic disorder (BDD), a mental *disorder* characterized by imagined ugliness. As you can tell by reading Jennifer's description, BDD is much more extreme than normal appearance concerns. BDD is also a psychiatric *diagnosis*, a label that mental health providers use to classify a disorder on the basis of its features. The *Diag-*

nostic and Statistical Manual of Mental Disorders (the current version is called the DSM-IV), published by the American Psychiatric Association, is a guide used by mental health professionals around the world to make diagnostic decisions. It describes all the important features of the mental health problems that are currently known.

To be diagnosed with BDD according to the DSM-IV, you would have to be preoccupied by a perceived appearance flaw that is either nonexistent or so small that only you view it as a problem, to the point that you're quite distressed by it or your daily functioning is disrupted. The professional making the diagnosis would also have to rule out other disorders as causes of these symptoms.

Some people with BDD acknowledge that their view of their appearance may be inaccurate and that they're blowing things out of proportion. "I know I'm not ugly," explained one of my patients. "I just can't stop thinking that my arms are too short. I'm a perfectionist, you know. I just wish I could stop beating myself up for my flaws." However, nearly half of all BDD sufferers hold their negative beliefs about their appearance with absolute certainty, despite what everyone else tells them. In those cases the evaluating practitioner should consider whether they also have what is called delusional disorder, somatic type. The degree to which those with BDD are convinced of their appearance-related beliefs determines whether they should be diagnosed with BDD alone or with BDD and delusional disorder.

Severity is an important measure of whether someone has BDD. If the preoccupation with a flaw does not cause real distress or impairment, it probably won't be diagnosed as BDD. People with this disorder are tormented by their concerns and, as we've seen, often have trouble keeping a job or a social life, because they can't tolerate the gaze and perceived judgment of others, or because the rituals they perform to improve their appearance take up so much of their time. In its most severe cases, BDD disables its sufferers and keeps them housebound for many years. The rate of alcohol and drug problems in those with BDD is close to 50%. The rate of suicide attempts is also relatively high, around 22–24%.

Concern about appearance is a symptom of some other psychiatric disorders too, so it's important for BDD to be diagnosed by someone who understands the distinctions. Those with anorexia nervosa, for example, are certainly concerned about their looks, but anorexia is always associated with severely disturbed eating behavior, and the appearance preoccupation focuses exclusively on weight. Still, BDD symptoms often mimic those of other disorders, which can easily lead to misdiagnosis and inaccurate treatment. Also, some similar conditions can co-occur with BDD symptoms but require separate treatment. The Appendix, "The Relationship of BDD to Other Disorders," sums up the differences and similarities of which you should be aware. For more detailed information on this topic, I recommend *The Broken Mirror* (see the Resources at the end of the book).

Just like normal appearance concerns, BDD usually begins during adolescence. It tends to be chronic, often lasting for many years without major improvement or relief. BDD occurs about as often in men as it does in women. Reports about individuals with BDD come from many different countries, including Germany, Japan, Russia, and England. Although no large-scale studies have been done on the rate of body dissatisfaction among various racial and ethnic groups, in my experience, these problems affect everyone, regardless of ethnic, economic, or education background. BDD used to be considered a rare disorder, but recent estimates range from 0.7% in the community to 13.0% in college students.

Do You Have BDD?

As I said in the Preface, you can benefit from the methods described in this book whether you have mild concerns that get in the way of a good life or you suffer from BDD. But it helps to have an idea of the severity of your problem before you tackle it, so answering the questions on page 10 may provide a clue as to whether you have BDD. A diagnosis can be made only by a qualified professional (the Resources at the end of this book will give you some guidance for finding a therapist or psychiatrist).

If you answer "yes" to *all* of the questions in the box on the next page and your primary problem isn't related to unusual eating habits, you probably suffer from BDD. If your BDD is severely distressing or impairing, you should not use this book alone, but rather as an adjunct to regular visits with a clinician. Also, if you have any doubts about your ability or willingness to try self-help, please find a qualified clinician with experience in treating body image concerns like BDD.

If you answer "yes" to only *some* of the questions about BDD, you might have milder appearance concerns, but this book might still be useful to you. Sometimes people with BDD are absolutely convinced that they look disfigured, when they actually look fine. In this case, they might doubt that they have BDD, and might even say that all the avoidance behaviors and appearance rituals are justified to protect themselves from teasing. If you fall into this group of people, it can be difficult to determine on your own whether you have BDD. To get around this issue, I included the question (1c) about how other people evaluate your appearance. If you are unsure how to answer it, you may want to consider meeting with a trained clinician.

Are You Worried Enough to Do Something about It?

This is the $64,000 question. Making changes in your behavior and your outlook can be an overwhelming prospect, and it's tough to know before you try

Clues to the Presence of BDD

1. a. Do you dislike the way any part(s) of your body (for example, your skin, hair, nose, or genitals) look?

    b. Do you think about your appearance for more than 1 hour per day?

    c. Do you think your worries about your appearance are excessive, or have others told you that you look OK and you just worry too much about your looks?

2. a. Do you engage in any behaviors intended to check on, hide, or fix your appearance (for example, mirror checking, comparing yourself to others, excessive grooming behaviors, or asking others about your appearance)?

    b. Do you avoid any places, people, or activities because of your appearance concerns (for example, do you avoid bright lights, mirrors, dating, or parties)?

3. Do your appearance-related thoughts or behaviors cause you a lot of anxiety, sadness, or shame?

4. Do you have problems with your work, school, family, or friends because of your appearance concerns?

Do You Suffer from Depression?

Everyone feels down at times; this is normal. But if your depression lasts for extended periods of time and causes significant distress, you might have a problem that requires treatment. If you think you might suffer from depression, please take a look at the following symptoms associated with depression:

- Feeling sad, down, or irritable for weeks or even longer
- Diminished interest or pleasure in your hobbies or typical activities
- Feeling tired in spite of lack of activity, low energy
- Increased or decreased appetite, with significant weight gain or weight loss
- Difficulty sleeping, waking up too early in the morning, or sleeping more than usual
- Feeling slowed down, or feeling restless or fidgety, diminished ability to make decisions or difficulty concentrating
- Feeling worthless, guilty, or hopeless
- Thoughts of suicide or death

Up to three-quarters of those with BDD are also depressed. So if you have been diagnosed with BDD or think you might have it, and you are also experiencing several of these symptoms of depression, talk to a qualified health care professional.

---

whether you're prepared to undertake the effort. With my patients, awareness of the scope and depth of the problem often fuels motivation. So, before you decide how to use this book, take a closer look at your own appearance concerns. I'll provide plenty of examples of others to serve as comparisons. If you begin to see yourself more and more in these portraits, you might find yourself motivated to get back the good life that your body image disturbance has taken from you.

What Are You Worried About?

Appearance obsessions can come in many forms. Whereas some people dislike just one body part, others are concerned about several. Some people worry about certain body parts for a while, then focus on new ones. Other people realize they look average but are still tormented, because they'd like to look perfect. Still others think they look disgusting and yearn to look normal.

What bothers *you* when you look in the mirror? Your appearance concerns could focus on any body part—nose, teeth, ears, head shape or size, fingers, legs, buttocks, feet, genitals, body build, and so on. Concerns with the face are among the most common.

The Face You Show the World

People are often preoccupied with their facial skin. They worry that their skin is too red or pale, or that their pores are too large. Other people are concerned about blemishes, pimples, "bumps," "zits," "spots," scars, freckles, lines, and wrinkles. All Susan can think of are the freckles on her face and arms. She tries to cover them up with clothing and wears long sleeves, even when it's 80 degrees out. People who have concerns about pimples or blemishes often try to correct them by spending a lot of time picking at their skin, often using small tools such as pins or tweezers. The problem with skin picking is that it can lead to actual scarring, which then causes even more worries.

Bad Hair Days—Every Day

Hair concerns are also very common. People are concerned that their hair is thinning or their hairline is receding. They may be worried that their hair is coarse, too curly or too straight, the wrong color, or asymmetrical. Maisha is obsessed with her hair. If it isn't right, she gets very upset and combs it over and over again. She once got in a car accident because she kept checking her hair in the rearview mirror while driving through a busy intersection.

Haircuts are usually very difficult for people with hair concerns. Brenda once told me: "Each haircut is a major procedure. I need to discuss every step in detail with my hairdresser. But no matter how hard my hairdresser tries, my hair is too long, too short, or not symmetrical. It is never right." Convinced his hair is thinning, Steve wears a hat all the time, even indoors, and spends a lot of time searching the Internet for hair-replacement procedures. Frank really dislikes the hair on his neck and spends large amounts of money on laser treatment and electrolysis. He even feels he could never move to another city, because he isn't sure he would be able to find adequate electrolysis elsewhere. Despite all of his efforts to remove his neck hair, he's convinced people are staring at him: "Girls laugh about me. I really think this is unfair—I don't laugh about them when they don't look perfect." Because she thinks she has too much facial hair, Anne avoids sitting under bright lights and never rolls down the windows in her car. She is often late to work because she "loses track of time" while tweezing her hair before leaving the house. Anne hates it when her boyfriend touches her face, because she's concerned that "he might think I'm growing a beard."

Pig Noses and Crooked Teeth

"I hate my nose," says Sean. "I look like a pig. I will never find a girlfriend—unless I get a nose job. . . ." Nose concerns are a widespread complaint among people with a poor body image. Like Sean, they daydream about plastic surgery. But, like Katie from the beginning of the chapter, they are often disappointed

---

A Warning about Weight Concerns

There is some overlap of symptoms between BDD and eating disorders. Please note that if you have not only weight concerns that resemble the symptoms of BDD but also disturbed eating patterns, the program in this book will not be enough to help, and you should seek professional help without delay. It is possible that you have an eating disorder. Eating disorders are serious illnesses with a high mortality rate.

---

with the results and end up angry at their surgeon if they actually do go under the knife.

Naja hates her "crooked" teeth, pronouncing them "really grotesque," and avoids smiling, often looking down or covering her mouth with her hands when she speaks.

Does Size Matter?

Americans love big sex organs. No one is immune to the widespread messages regarding the importance of size, whether it's the penis for men or breasts for women. Naturally, many feel inadequately equipped. Dan considers his "short" penis "unmanly" and after padding his pants for years is currently considering surgery as a more permanent solution.

Some people are overly concerned with their overall body build or height. At 5'7", Harry feels "like a dwarf" and can hardly tolerate being around tall women. Eric is preoccupied with his muscles. Although he already has a V-shaped torso, he strives for "wider shoulders and bigger biceps." He lifts weights every day and often gets into arguments with his girlfriend, because he prefers lifting to spending time with her. "She tells me I look great and that she loves me as I am. But I want to look stronger and manlier. That's how I got so obsessed with lifting."

How Do You Feel about the Way You Look?

People with body image disturbances are often ruled by how they feel about their appearance. You're likely to feel embarrassed in social situations. Feeling self-conscious and shameful about your defect may lead you to avoid certain people, places, or situations. Doing so is problematic on its own, because you miss out on things you would otherwise enjoy. In addition, though, everyone needs social contact, and not participating in social activities will leave you feeling sad and lonely. Also keep in mind that if you don't go to certain events, you'll never find out whether your horrific predictions that people will stare at your defect will actually come true. If you had gone, perhaps nobody would have noticed or cared. You might feel frustrated about spending so much time and money on beauty rituals, only to find out that it's a never-ending pattern: No matter what you do, you're still dissatisfied with your looks. If your self-esteem is low, you might feel envious when you focus on the appearance of others, because you notice only what they have that you lack. You might even feel intensely jealous or insecure in relationships. You might feel nervous and confused when you get a compliment. Your mood, along with the way you see yourself, might be like riding on a roller coaster. When you feel that you look good, you might be happy and relatively self-confident, but if anything triggers your appearance concerns (like meeting someone who looks better or just having a pimple), your self-esteem might be shattered. You become convinced that the only way to feel better is to look better. This is one of the fundamental beliefs behind body image disturbance.

What Are Your Thoughts and Beliefs about Your Appearance?

If you have severe appearance concerns, you might think others notice your flaw and are repelled by it. You worry that anyone you talk to will look at your defect, and you'll then feel ashamed of it. You're suspicious of compliments. You may even believe others are talking and laughing about your supposed flaw, as Reid did, when he walked out of a store and noticed a couple of girls looking in his direction and giggling. He immediately thought, *"They must be laughing about my thinning hair!"* (If he couldn't stop thinking about his hair, he reasoned, how could anyone else?) And even though he had no evidence to support this assumption, Reid felt sad and discouraged.

Many people also assume that the defect they're sure they have is a visible manifestation of some character flaw. Personal worth and physical appearance become commingled and confused. Jean is a petite, pretty 18-year-old with a hook at the end of her nose. Her friends don't even notice and just think of her as beautiful, but Jean believes her nose makes her look "really ugly and mean." With tears in her eyes, and avoiding eye contact, she says, "How I am on the inside, that's how I look on the outside: bad and repulsive. . . . I don't think I'll ever find a boyfriend or get married because of my looks. Who'd be attracted to a mean, ugly witch?"

Many people with body image disturbances believe they'll end up alone and unloved. You'd never know it to look at her, but Li Ming is extremely concerned with blemishes on her skin and excessive facial hair, especially on her eyebrows. She recently started dating Rich, a really nice guy. But she's afraid of spending a full night with him. "I've always been self-conscious about my skin and my eyebrows. We've been dating for a few months now, but he's never seen me without makeup. If he stayed over, I would have to take my makeup off at night, and then I would have to put it back on in the morning before he wakes up. I usually also spend quite a bit of time plucking my eyebrows and penciling them in so they look just right. I won't let anyone see me before my appearance is acceptable. On bad days, when I feel my skin is broken out, it can take me a couple of hours to get ready. I just don't know what to do. If Rich notices how much time I take to get ready in the morning, he'll think I'm nuts. But I can't let him see me with bushy eyebrows or without makeup. If he'd known what I really look like, he'd never have gone out with me in the first place. To be honest, it makes me feel guilty that he's never seen the 'real' me. It's like I'm leading him on. But I don't want to lose him. If he sees how ugly I really am, he'll break up with me. I feel I'm stuck in this awful situation, and I don't see a way to resolve it. I don't think I'll ever be able to be happy unless my appearance changes."

If you hold similar beliefs about the relationship of appearance and self-worth, you're really in trouble when you think your appearance is imperfect. As a result, you might feel sad or anxious and start to avoid social activities. Or you might engage in all kinds of activities to fix whatever you consider the appearance problem to be.

What Rituals Do You Perform in the Name of Beauty?

Paula spends a lot of time reading beauty magazines, buying flattering clothes and cosmetics, having her hair styled and colored, and her nails done, and getting makeovers. She can easily spend several hours a day on these rituals, but, at best, they provide only temporary relief. "I always have to try to look my best," she explains. "I just don't want to be caught off guard. What if someone made a negative comment about my appearance or teased me? I couldn't handle that!" So she never goes out without makeup and perfectly styled hair, and taking those measures does ease the anxiety of going out in public. That's why she's not ready to give up her rituals, despite the fact that she's fed up with always trying to know about the latest makeup techniques and products, and new hairstyles.

Do you believe the only way to change your negative feelings about your body is to change your body? Do you spend a lot of time or money trying to improve your looks? If so, you're not alone. Most people with body image problems engage in repetitive behaviors intended to check, improve, or hide whatever they're concerned about.

Mirrors are maddening to Kelly, who says she can't walk past one without checking a small scar right under her nose. Judy can't leave the house until her makeup perfectly disguises the fact that she looks "really old and unattractive" because "My eyes often look so tired, and I have lots of wrinkles around them. And my lips have gotten thinner and thinner over the years." John spends a lot of time in front of the mirror trying to camouflage blemishes on his cheeks with a spot stick—"like a girl," he says with self-disgust.

Other people engage in excessive grooming, such as combing, cutting, or styling their hair. Richard spends a lot of time before and during work combing and recombing his hair to cover his bald spot—to the point that he's worried his office mate thinks he must be lazy because he spends so much time away from his desk.

Adam works out every day, often for a couple of hours at a time. His friends admire his dedication and discipline. What they don't know is that Adam takes steroids and is always anxious about looking weak and sickly. His personal trainer has already told him to cut back on his workouts or he'll injure himself. If Adam misses a workout, though, he feels lazy and ashamed. On top of over-exercising, some men with poor body image overconsume protein shakes and abuse anabolic steroids. In his research on body builders, Dr. Harrison Pope has found that 9% suffer from what he calls "muscle dysmorphia." Dr. Pope describes this fear of being weak and small as a reverse form of anorexia nervosa: Whereas anorexic patients may diet excessively because they fear getting fat, individuals with muscle dysmorphia may exercise excessively or abuse steroids because of a fear of looking too thin. Some are so ashamed of their thin arms that they wind up wearing long sleeves even in the summer. Others are so eager to look big and muscular that they pad their clothes. Still others go so far as to have plastic surgery. Tyler wanted to have the biggest pecs possible, without spending several hours a week at the gym, so he opted for a $3,000 procedure in which rubber implants were inserted under his pectoral muscles. Unfortunately, Tyler isn't happy with the results, because the surgery didn't help him win back his unfaithful partner. Now he is considering cheek implants. For some people, surgery seems to be addictive, and they keep going back over and over again for more, without any long-term improvement of their body image.

Other people may not take as drastic a measure as surgery to improve their appearance, but they remove imperfections on their own either by tweezing or picking their skin. Eva has picked at her face since she was a teenager. Now she also picks at her back and arms. She picks at whiteheads and blackheads. When she came to my office, I could not see any acne-related problems, but she had the telltale signs of someone with a skin-picking problem: little red picking marks covering her entire face. "I just have to get this disgusting white stuff out! My face looks really ugly with all these bumps on it! I know it sounds weird, but I actually feel good while I'm picking at my skin. I feel like I'm cleaning it. But after I'm done, I beat myself up for the mess I've made. My face usually looks really red, and the bumps seem swollen." Eva admits that she usually starts gently and tells herself that she will just take care of this one pimple, but then the habit gets out of control, and she picks for hours. "I think my intentions are good, and I try to improve my appearance, but somehow the outcome is always bad because I overdo it. . . . Once I get started, I just cannot stop!"

Most appearance rituals don't directly affect your relationships, because you can do them by yourself. However, you may include others in your appearance rituals by asking them over and over again what they think of your new haircut, or whether they notice a pimple. A patient of mine, Monica, was predominantly concerned with her pale skin. She had two ways of carrying out her rituals, either by checking the mirror herself or by asking her husband what he thought of her skin. When I worked with her in behavior therapy, we quickly conquered the mirror checking. Monica gradually decreased the checking each week until she finally reached a normal level. However, her negative thoughts related to her appearance and her urges to check the mirror were not improving. This surprised me. After a few weeks, her husband Henry joined us for a treatment session. Henry told me that Monica asked him about her skin about six or seven times per day. She would even ask him to look at her face in different lighting and from different angles. Not surprisingly, Henry was quite fed up with his wife's quest for reassurance. When I asked Henry why he went along with her requests, he explained that this was actually easier than "fighting with her about it." He was not aware that by trying to help her, he was actually making her problem worse by participating in a ritual.

There is another behavior, in addition to reassurance seeking, that might affect your relationships. Do you compare your appearance to that of others? When you look at other people, you probably focus only on those body parts of other people you wish you could have. When you look at yourself in the mirror, you likely notice only the body parts with which you're unhappy. This leads to a distorted body image: You don't see how you really look; rather, you see what you consider the worst about yourself. This way you always lose the appearance competition.

Even though engaging in the rituals just described seems like a good way to ward off the anxiety people feel about their appearance, it rarely eliminates all of the insecurity that those with body dissatisfaction feel. If that's true for you, you probably also avoid certain situations that you would probably enjoy if your body image were better.

What Are You Avoiding These Days?

Elvira, a 34-year-old salesperson, did fine selling products over the phone. However, when she got promoted, she was asked to make sales pitches one-on-one or even to groups. This caused a big problem. Being seen by strangers made her extremely nervous. All she could think of was "They're looking at my skin." She was sure that others were staring at her pimples. Her heart beat rapidly in sales situations, and she started sweating. Elvira tried to avoid these situations as much as possible, which led to her losing lots of money. She also started spending even more money than she used to on expensive skin care products designed to correct her imagined skin problem. Ultimately, she asked to return to her lower paying phone position.

As we've seen, many people with a poor body image avoid social situations, but some adopt more subtle avoidance strategies, such as not sitting under a bright light.

Sex has always been something of a problem for Samantha. When in her 20s, she was concerned that she was not thin enough, that her thighs looked too big. Now, in her 40s, Samantha worries about the wrinkles on her forehead and the crow's-feet around her eyes. Married for 13 years, she has a good relationship with her husband but is so self-conscious about the signs of aging she sees in herself that it's affecting her sex life: "Now we make love only in the dark. My husband would really like me to leave the lights on, but I just don't like this anymore. If I keep the light on, all I can think of is what he might be thinking of my appearance." Samantha is so busy worrying about her appearance that it's difficult for her to experience the positive feelings that usually accompany sex. Although she knows her husband loves her and the way she looks, she rejects her own body.

You might also experience subtle behaviors such as avoidance of eye contact or disengaging from uncomfortable situations by daydreaming or distracting yourself. If you have a severe body image problem, it is quite likely that you have a troublesome relationship with mirrors. Caught between wanting to avoid your reflection and wanting to fix it, you might alternate between episodes of mirror avoidance and mirror checking.

Camouflaging is also an avoidance behavior. Many people hide the perceived defect with makeup, hair, their body position, or clothes. Virginia always wears a hat or bandana to hide what she considers her protruding ears. Timmy wears baseball caps to conceal his thinning hair. Nancy slouches, preferring poor posture to standing up straight, because she thinks she's too tall.

Clearly, avoidance causes you to miss out on things you'd probably enjoy otherwise, but it can also narrow your life increasingly. Avoiding an activity or situation reduces your confidence in your ability to handle that activity or situation the next time.

In the following chapters, we'll look at several strategies that will help you feel more secure about your appearance. Together we'll develop a program that will progress in a gradual manner, and we'll break the cycles maintaining body image concerns. You'll learn to overcome your problems by changing self-defeating thoughts, setting realistic goals to reduce frenzied appearance rituals, and creating exercises that will prevent you from hiding your appearance. You will learn how to conquer your avoidance behaviors and beauty compulsions in a step-by-step fashion. Together we'll work toward a peaceful relationship between you and your body.

Chapter 2

"Why Do I Feel
So Unattractive?"

Did you recognize any of the people described in Chapter 1? When you started reading, you may have felt a sense of relief that your appearance concern is different from the concerns of Peter, Emily, Ahmed, and Katie. Maybe the way you feel about your nose or your legs, your skin or your hair, your height or your bone structure, is perfectly normal after all. But if you've gotten this far, most likely it's because you began to see yourself in some of the behaviors and feelings that people with BDD and milder body image disturbances seem to have in common. Fortunately, this recognition should also bring a sense of relief. What you do or avoid because of the way you feel about your looks may be out of proportion, but it's a problem shared by many. Now the question is how you got here.

People with body image disturbances often get so wrapped up in their beauty rituals and avoidance gambits that they can hardly remember life without them. Stepping back and looking at similar patterns in others, as we did in Chapter 1, can give you just the distance you need to begin to wonder why you feel so unattractive. How did worry about your appearance begin to take over your life? Why are you so much more concerned about how you look than are other people you know? The answer is not likely to be simple. Our understanding of the causes of body image disturbance is far from complete. We do know, however, that a complex mix of environmental and biological factors may come into play, including messages from the media, the legacy of family culture, and the influence of peers, personality traits, and the mechanics and chemistry of the brain.

How Our Environment Creates Body Image Problems

Andrea religiously reads fashion magazines and is always trying to stay up to date on the latest hairstyles, makeup, diets, exercise, and clothing. She admits that looking at perfect-looking women makes her feel bad, "but I still cut their pictures out of the magazine and put them on the wall," she says. "This keeps me motivated to improve my appearance!" Andrea is driven by two misconceptions that bombard us everywhere today: that "perfect" looks are both desirable and attainable.

Beauty: Today's Holy Grail

TV and the fashion magazines keep telling us there is a perfect look we should try to achieve, and these messages can have a strong impact on our body image. You, just like everybody else, are flooded by messages about the advantages of looking beautiful. In advertisements and movies, you are told, sometimes directly, other times in a roundabout way, that admiration, success, power, intelligence, friends, fun, and romance are all related to beauty. You've probably also learned that unattractive people are failures: They are laughable, lazy, dangerous, mad, stupid, or morally reprehensible. The mean characters in shows for children—witches, nasty stepmothers, monsters—are usually not only evil but also ugly and deformed.

For thousands of years, people have applied cosmetics, and sprinkled and sprayed their bodies. The desire to enhance physical beauty is nothing new. But movies, TV, and now the Internet have encouraged us to take this desire to new extremes—in some cases, dangerous ones. Everywhere we turn, print and electronic media expose us over and over to the beautiful few, leaving us with the false impression that millions of men and women are practically perfect looking. Our assumptions about what's normal naturally might have changed.

Of course, we are seeing not millions of perfectly beautiful people but a virtual handful of models who appear in different guises throughout the media. And according to my colleague Nancy Etcoff,* models' proportions are so unusual that they could be considered "genetic freaks." In addition, many of us are unaware that we see only a model's perfect part. There are shoe models, leg models, hand models, lip models. . . . The tall supermodels could never be shoe models, because their feet are too big. The "perfect" foot is small, about a size 6.

I once took a bus in New York City and overheard a young woman sitting behind me talk about her glamorous career as an underwear model. Of course, I was curious to see how she looked. When I finally turned around, I was quite amazed at how plain her face was. I would never have noticed her in a crowd.

---

*Nancy Etcoff, *Survival of the Prettiest: The Science of Beauty* (Anchor Books, 1999).

But then it struck me that her breasts, stomach, and legs seemed close to perfect, and that was all that mattered for her job. Often the media do not show us just a part of one person, but computer-merged images consisting of body parts of many people. One model might contribute the face; another, the body; and a third, the hair. Hollywood uses body-doubles because someone's beautiful face looks even better if it is matched with somebody else's great body.

You may find this hard to believe, but the beautiful people on TV and in magazines don't really exist. They are no more real than the dinosaurs in *Jurassic Park*. Even if you just see the picture of one model, what you probably don't think about is that this model has spent hours with professional makeup artists, hairstylists, and clothes designers just for one picture. The model might also have had plastic surgery and probably follows a rigidly controlled exercise and diet program. Just for one photograph, he or she is put in the most pleasing position and lighting possible. After pictures are taken, artists go to work to provide fake color, airbrush, and digital imaging. In the end, everything looks much better than nature ever intended.

A number of research studies have shown that people are less satisfied with their own looks after seeing beautiful models in fashion magazines, and it's no wonder. Greta tells me that she gets frustrated when she reads women's magazines. "All the girls in there are so pretty. And I just feel like crying when I see their pictures. It makes me mad. And then there is all this advice on how to look better: fashion advice, all these masks and makeup tips, and stuff like that. I keep trying it, but it just doesn't really cut it. Why can't I be pretty? I hate everything about my looks. I look so blah and boring. And then my hair and eyes are dark, and I am short. I want to be blonde and tall. I am so envious when I see these pretty girls. People tell me that I am nice and smart and a really good friend. But I don't care about that. I want to be pretty."

Fortunately, there are signs that media messages about how people—at least women—are supposed to look are beginning to shift toward realism. In the decade before this book was published, advertisers started to make an effort to portray women in nonstereotypical ways, and by 2005, Americans saw everything from a Nike campaign that started with a woman proclaiming, "My butt is big," to Dove ads and billboards showing women in a variety of sizes, and showing wrinkles and other natural signs of aging, to a Body Shop ad that paired a Rubenesque plastic doll with the statement, "There are 3 billion women who don't look like supermodels and only 8 who do." These evolving messages, combined with greater awareness of the damage that overemphasis on appearance can cause, and greater visibility of women with long lists of occupational and other accomplishments to their credit, may account for the fact that body image may no longer be worsening over time. Dr. Thomas Cash, in a study that examined changes in body image from 1983 to 2001, found that nonblack women's appearance dissatisfaction increased until the early or mid-1990s, after which *body image evaluations improved* in both nonblack and black women. Interestingly, investment in their appearance for the women surveyed had also decreased over time (they were now placing less importance on being attractive and attending to their looks, and spending less time in appearance management behaviors). For men, Dr. Cash found that body image was stable over the 19-year period. So, although body image disturbance remains a significant problem, at least one study has seen signs that the trend is changing in a positive direction.

Nevertheless, listening to the majority of media sources today may make us feel like we have to find the right product, wear the right clothes, work out (with the correct equipment, of course), and get plastic surgery. After we've done all this, happiness and romance will come automatically—right? Maybe not. If you believe in these messages by the beauty industry, they can drive you into a frenzy to improve your looks. If you choose to do nothing about your appearance, you might feel unattractive and lazy. You might also feel scrutinized and insecure in social situations. After all, other people must have high standards too, and maybe they will find you wanting.

So we believe a "perfect" appearance is worth striving for, and some of us feel obligated to pursue it. In many cases, the groundwork was laid when we were too young to question the messages we were receiving.

Starting Young: The Toy Industry

The toy industry does its part to convince us that there's a very high standard of beauty to be met and that we should try to meet it. When I recently surfed the Internet looking for a doll for my daughter, I came across Makeup Mindy, a best-seller that comes with a makeup kit and teaches little girls age 3 and older the rite of applying cosmetics to face, nails, and hair. It didn't take long for me to realize that Makeup Mindy is just one of many similar dolls, a fact confirmed in a survey conducted by the Renfrew Center, where clinicians found that 90% of the toys and dolls surveyed for girls ages 2–10 years emphasize applying makeup and jewelry, shopping for clothes, or dating.

If you grew up playing with Barbies, you know the kind of ideal that dolls can promote. Modeled after the German doll "Lilli," a sex toy for men, Barbie has become a symbol of sexism. Inez, a very attractive, very athletic patient with (dyed) long blonde hair and concerns about her skin and weight, told me: "To me, my Barbie dolls were beautiful. I wanted to look like them. It was not an unrealistic aspiration in my mind. My dolls all had wardrobes of clothes for all occasions—some matched my own outfits! Between us, my sister and I must have had twenty or more Barbie dolls alone. At the time, I didn't think about their small waists, large chests, beautiful blonde hair, and sparkling blue eyes. But I do remember at one point I had the impression that when I grew up, I would look just as beautiful as the Barbie doll, because that was what I imagined an adult woman was supposed to look like. I guess I thought my hair would just naturally change from brown to blonde (maybe this didn't happen naturally, but I still wish . . .) and I would develop a body just like hers. After all, I thought that was just the way life progressed—from baby, to child, Barbie-like bombshell, mother, and old lady."

Barbie has grown thinner and thinner over the years and has been blamed for the emergence of eating disorders in girls and women. And Barbie is not alone. Over the past 20 years, the action toys marketed to target young boys also have evolved. The current GI Joe is much more muscular than his original counterpart. Buzz Lightyear, Iron Man, and Batman all have the bulging muscles of bodybuilders. Concerned about their increasingly unrealistic body proportions, psychiatrists are now warning about the impact that action figures might have on the body image of boys.

One of my patients once remarked that "the lesson of accepting all sizes and shapes would be an important value to instill while children are still impressionable and open-minded" and wondered, as many other women I've talked to have wondered, why the toy industry hasn't come up with more "real"-looking dolls, with proportions more like those of the average woman or man, so that when children are older, they become more accepting people. None of my patients knew that in 1991, a company called High Self-Esteem Toys had developed a rival for Barbie. Her name was "Happy to Be Me," and initially it looked like she might be the answer to the complaint of so many women. She had wider hips and waist, shorter neck and legs, and her feet were flat and molded for sensible shoes. Happy made international headlines when she was first introduced, but 14 years later, she is nowhere to be found. And even the phone number for High Self-Esteem Toys is no longer listed.

All good intentions aside, Happy was apparently a sales bust. In contrast, dolls and action figures that represent an unattainable ideal—and an undesirable one—are best-selling toys year after year. Why? Because children apparently prefer role models with glamorous outfits and spectacular beauty. This should be no surprise. After all, they see the same ads, movies, and TV shows that adults do.

Good Looks: You Can Have Them If You Really Try (and Buy)

All of the Barbies and similar toys send a doubly dangerous message: Not only is being pretty important but also appearance can be improved by using makeup or buying the right clothes. In the process, they stereotype women and leave little room for creativity or imagination. They instill the myth that perfection is attainable in the most impressionable minds, and it's a myth that for many people lingers into adulthood.

Inez found herself making different efforts every year to look more like the doll she thought she would grow up to resemble. "In fourth grade I copied some exercises from my mom's magazine word-for-word into my notebook, because I felt that I needed to start working out. I didn't like the way my legs looked. Or, for my junior prom, I had searched everywhere I could to find a corset to make me look skinnier. I never found one, mostly because I was too embarrassed to ask for it. Just like I was embarrassed to tear pages for exercising out of my mom's magazine. . . . I was ashamed I did not look like the Barbie doll already. I was full of ideals that could never be attained, and I think that doll is partly to blame."

Unfortunately, the kids targeted by these toy makers are too young to understand that perfect bodies, perfect hair, and perfect skin are unattainable for most people. These types of toys, combined with daily commercial messages about beauty, can promote thinking that sets the stage for endless hours of makeup applications, clothes shopping, cosmetic surgeries, and excessive exercise.

Again, people have always primped and preened to a certain extent. But our devotion to such perfection-seeking efforts has grown exponentially over the last several decades. Whereas rouged cheeks and darkened eyelids were still considered signs of female vice in the 19th century, 80–90% of adult American women were using lipstick and about 67% were using rouge by 1948. High-powered advertising was fundamental to this change. Over the years, the beauty industry has developed elaborate campaigns around enticing product names. Ads have been illustrated with flawless models, and consumption has become essential to achieve perfect appearance. Beauty promises and personality changes have become strangely intertwined. Ponds, for example, promised that their product would produce a "warm, Inner You." The beauty industry also segmented the market, and the fashionable face changes every season, which also compels the consumer to buy new products continuously to keep their looks up to date.

What do these messages by the beauty industry do to people like you and me? Whenever you read a fashion magazine, you probably feel like you have a mountain of self-improvement work ahead of you. Every inch of your body needs to be perfumed, or treated with lotions or sprays of one kind or another. Your teeth need to be straightened and whitened, your eyebrows plucked, your eyelashes shaded, your lips thickened, and your thighs thinned. Not only do these measures need to be taken, but they *will* produce perfection—if only you try hard enough and spend enough money. Currently in the United States, more money is invested in beauty than in education or social services. Indeed, we spend more money on personal care products than on reading material. According to statistics released by the American Society of Plastic Surgeons, 9.2 million cosmetic surgery procedures were performed in 2004, and $8.4 billon was spent on cosmetic surgery. Trending data show that cosmetic plastic surgery procedures increased by 700% from 1992 to 2004. Reality TV shows such as *Extreme Makeover* have raised the awareness for plastic surgery and make it look like it's no big deal to get multiple plastic surgery procedures at the same time. Cosmetic surgery is no longer just for the rich and famous; it has become a more acceptable procedure for regular folks as well.

Just a few years ago, my hair salon paired up with a plastic surgeon. Now customers can make an appointment for a haircut and a face-lift with one phone call.

Meanwhile, in the last 50 years, the beauty industry started targeting teenagers and children, as well as adults. Teen magazines, websites, and the MTV network are filled with ads for acne preparations and teen cosmetics. No doubt these marketing efforts will continue, or even increase, because they are apparently very effective.

Indeed, 13- to 19-year-old girls spend more than $9 billion a year on cosmetics, fragrances, and other beauty care products, according to Teenage Research Unlimited. Several of my patients have told me they started using makeup before they were 13 years old, a trend confirmed by a casual glance at virtually any American junior high school class today. Marketers are targeting young males, too. According to a report by Market Research.com, hair styling and coloring products have emerged as the fastest growing segments of the personal care market among teen and tween males.

Ironically, concurrent with the increase in cosmetic use over the last five or six decades has come an increase in body image concerns. As early as the 1930s, women were stating that advertising and related social appearance pressure had a negative effect on their self-esteem.

With all these beauty products and services available to us, we should be feeling better, not worse, about our looks, because now all of us can look pretty good. Unfortunately, "pretty good" is not good enough when what you're expecting is perfection.

If you are like me, you probably have neither the genes nor the time nor the money to achieve the perfect look that's portrayed in the various ads. However, seeing those images over and over distorts your idea of what is normal, or even what is possible. And this is true for most of us. No matter how old we are, we want to keep all our hair, have unlined faces, and maintain flat stomachs. Of course, there is nothing wrong with wanting to look attractive. But although some changes may be possible through cosmetic surgery or other beauty procedures, most of us will never reach society's ideal. This leaves us comparing ourselves against unrealistic standards. We set goals that we can never reach. And if we do not recognize this pattern, we may feel defective and ashamed.

Cultural Influences

Because the United States has been at the vanguard of modern marketing and the development of electronic media, preoccupation with appearance and striving for physical perfection have often been called strictly American preoccupations. However, case reports from all over the world indicate that the similarities across cultures are striking, and that BDD is not simply a Western problem. For example, across cultures, the age of onset is similar, and so is the presence of beauty rituals (e.g., mirror checking) and the high rates of depression and anxiety. Again, this may be a product of the pervasiveness of the media all over the world today. Where we do see differences is in the expression of BDD symptoms. Excessive appearance concerns with eyelids seem to be more common among Asians, which perhaps reflects the overall trend that eyelid surgery is the fastest growing type of plastic surgery in the Asian community. In general, individuals of different ethnicities try to transform themselves to fit a stereotypical Caucasian and "all American" beauty standard.

I've also seen several patients who, concerned with their "Jewish" nose, underwent rhinoplasty, a cosmetic surgery for the nose. A Hispanic man recently told me that he is very concerned with his "Spanish" looks ever since he moved to the United States. He was concerned that he would not fit in and would always be seen and treated like a foreigner. Another patient of mine moved from Germany to the United States. He had been very socially anxious and somewhat concerned about his weight before immigrating, but after living here for a few weeks, he became extremely preoccupied with his teeth. He told me that in contrast to Germans, most Americans had perfect teeth. Because two of his teeth were crooked, he felt like people were staring at him. This made him so anxious that he looked down or covered his mouth while talking.

We are all exposed to cultural influences, the mass media marketing the beauty industry, and the production of perfect-figure toys. But not everyone is affected by them equally; therefore, other factors must also play a role in the development of body image problems. Vulnerability factors, such as low self-esteem, must be present before we can be influenced by a TV ad or a picture in a magazine. Very powerful and early influences include the family one grows up in, teasing from peers as children, and, in some cases, physical or sexual abuse.

Family Members and Peers

Your beliefs about yourself and the world around you start to form early in childhood. Because your parents are such an integral part of your life, they play an important role in shaping your self-concept. Did your parents stress the importance of appearance when you were young, communicating that good looks are important to being loved and accepted? Some parents express this attitude directly; others do so indirectly. Some parents invest a lot of time, money, and energy in their own looks, passing on appearance concerns by example. Often it turns out that these parents themselves have been struggling with a poor body image. They might even have had plastic surgery. Other parents instill the idea that looks are paramount simply by going on and on about clothes, looks, and fashion in their daily conversation.

Still other parents spend a disproportionate amount of time ensuring that their children look attractive, either by being outright critical of their children's appearance or by taking excessive pride in a child's good looks and spending a lot of time and energy trying to highlight them. Many parents are not able just to accept their children's bodies. Others may have good intentions: All they want is to arm their children to compete in our appearance-conscious society. But, in the process, they get children into the habit of paying a lot of attention to how they look.

Yolanda, a young Latino woman, came to her first therapy appointment with her mother, Maria. The two looked more like sisters than mother and daughter. Their clothes were very expensive and their hair perfectly styled, with eyebrows plucked and makeup carefully applied. While Yolanda talked, her mother picked some lint off her jacket. Yolanda looked pretty, but she told me that she had a problem with excessive facial hair. I couldn't see any facial hair whatsoever, even though I really looked for it. Her eyes filled with tears when she told me that a few years ago, her brother had asked her teasingly, "Are you growing a beard?" Since then, she had been very self-conscious about her face. She checked the mirror a lot and spent an enormous amount of time plucking and bleaching her facial hair. Trying on makeup and different clothes before she left the house was another activity she dreaded and that took up a lot of her time. Her beauty rituals led to her being late for almost everything.

Yolanda also admitted that she was $13,000 in debt due to several cosmetic procedures. She had had Botox injections, dermabrasions, and liposuction. On top of that, over the past few months, she had gone shopping almost daily for clothes and beauty products. She needed to buy something new for every event, she said, whether it was an evening with friends, a therapy appointment, or a change in season. The shopping helped her feel good for a little while, but after a day or two, she would feel that her clothes looked old, worn, or ill-fitting. She was afraid others would think she had bad taste or came from a low social class, so she had to go out and buy something new. Yolanda had maxed out one of her credit cards and was close to the limit on another one, which scared her tremendously, because her job as a cashier did not pay well and she had no idea how she would be able to pay back what she owed.

Maria told me, "I am just so worried about her. She's so beautiful, but she doesn't seem to see it. I wonder if we did something wrong. My husband and I are very interested in fashion, and we are both trying to stay fit. But not in a bad way, you know? But, I don't know, maybe we put too much pressure on Yolanda. We have always encouraged her to make an effort to look good, but now she definitely goes overboard with it."

Igor's story was similar. His father was tall, muscular, and worked out a lot. As a child, Igor was underweight and his puberty started late, so his father got very concerned about his looks. He pressured Igor to participate in sports and was very critical when Igor's athletic performance was not near perfect. Igor also told me that he had had a "lazy" eye when he was a child. His brothers had teased him about it, and his parents took him to the best surgeons around the country to get the problem corrected. By the time I first saw him, both of his eyes worked fine and I could not even detect which one had had the problem. Nevertheless, Igor felt very self-conscious about his eye. Even in therapy sessions, Igor initially sat in such a way that I could see only his "good" eye.

When I met him, Igor was 31, tall, muscular, and a successful marketing manager at a major company. Although quite handsome, he was struggling with a poor body image. His self-esteem would plummet whenever he felt that he did not look good. Especially when a date didn't go as well as he had hoped, he assumed that he was not attractive enough. During these times, his father's comments caught up with him. "You look like a wimp. Eat more and work out." Then Igor would ask for reassurance regarding his eye or throw himself into an excessive exercise regimen in an attempt to feel better. Unfortunately, neither of these strategies worked long term.

Families that overvalue physical appearance can unwittingly contribute to a poor body image. As a result of growing up in a family where beauty is heavily emphasized, your self-esteem might be directly tied to your appearance. No matter how you look, you may constantly feel like you should be more attractive. Parents who have extremely high expectations, or are very critical in general, might also produce feelings of insecurity in a child; thus, a minor appearance flaw or an occasional comment about some appearance issue might be blown out of proportion. Mary Beth is now in her 40s, and although she looks much younger than her actual age, she "hates" her looks. She particularly dislikes her nose, and she thinks she is too fat. When she was a child, her sister called her "pig nose." Mary Beth told me: "My parents were very strict, and I had to be perfect at everything I did. No matter what it was—grades, clothes, behavior, appearance, you name it—I always felt like I was on display. I never felt like I was just a little kid who could play, be silly, get dirty, and all that. And when this other kid called me 'pig nose,' that did it. It really crushed me. I felt so ashamed that I was so defective and flawed, and I could not forget it. I still worry about my nose, and this happened over 30 years ago!"

If your parents were overly critical of your appearance or other characteristics, it's not too surprising that you might be just as hard on yourself as an adult. But your parents can also plant a more subtle suggestion that your appearance is deficient by withholding physical affection or by being physically or sexually abusive. "My father beat me a lot," Saskia, a 50-year-old woman with concerns about freckles told me, "for the smallest things. Of course, this was more common in those days, but nowadays you would call it abuse. To makes things worse, my mother never hugged me unless I was injured. Sometimes I fell on purpose, so that she would touch me and pick me up. But I think that her usually not touching made me feel there was something really disgusting about me or my body. I felt unacceptable, unlovable. My parents never told me that I looked nice or pretty, which might have something to do with my feeling unattractive, too." Of course, although abuse or neglect may be a risk factor, not everyone with such a history develops body image problems, nor has every person who has body image problems experienced trauma or abuse.

If you were teased as a child, the teasing probably had a negative impact on your body image, and you might still be thinking about it years later. Often siblings are the worst critics, but parents or peers might have teased you as well. Yolanda had been teased about facial hair several years before she consulted me. Although the hair was gone when I first saw her (if it had ever been there), the shame was not. Yolanda's brother considered his comments harmless teasing, but Yolanda considered them highly damaging to her confidence in her appearance. Indeed, researchers who investigated the effects of teasing found that it is related to body dissatisfaction.

Childhood experiences probably have a strong impact on your body image, and most people develop BDD when they are still relatively young. However, once you have a weak spot in the body image department, your day-to-day experiences will further determine how you think and feel about your looks. A partner who criticizes your appearance, for example, may have a devastating influence on your body image.

As you can see in these examples, human behavior can be affected significantly by external or environmental factors such as social messages and our relationships and interactions with other people. But it's also guided by internal influences such as personality.

Is It Just My Personality?

Does your personality play a role in your negative body image? Possibly it does. Your personality is a result of both genetic and environmental influences. In other words, it is not only determined by biological factors, such as heredity, but it is also molded by your upbringing and whatever happened to you over the course of your life—the social and familial influences we've just discussed.

We don't know very much about a possible link between different personality traits and appearance concerns. The people I work with certainly have all different kinds of personalities, but I recently completed a study showing that BDD patients as a group have elevated levels of perfectionism. Indeed, many of my patients describe themselves as perfectionistic and fearful of criticism and rejection. If you find that this is true for you—you'll find a self-test to give you a clue a little farther along—you can use the program in this book to get these traits under control, so they're not so harmful to you in the future.

Perfectionism

When I asked Peter, the lawyer introduced in Chapter 1, why appearance became so important to him, he replied, "I just have very high standards for myself. I always worked very hard, so that I had very good grades. Even as a kid, I wouldn't give up until I had all the answers on a test figured out. I went to really good schools, and I'd always try for a 100 on each test. If I got anything worse than an A or A plus, I was really disappointed. And I think it's just the same with my looks. I could look so much better. And I am not going to let my genes stop me from looking better."

In a survey of people with BDD, conducted by Dr. David Veale in the United Kingdom, 69% affirmed the belief, "I have to have perfection in my appearance." The problem with this attitude is that physical perfection does not exist. It is an illusion, just like the models on magazine covers. Albrecht Dürer once said, "There lives on earth no one beautiful person who could not be more beautiful." That's true. Everybody's looks could be improved if you look at them closely and critically enough. Just try it. Pick out a person who looks very nice at first glance in a public place. I did it just recently, when I was in the mall thinking about this book. I saw a young man, about 25, who looked very handsome at first glance. I kept looking, curious about whether I would find something that was not perfect. I found some blackheads around his nose. First I noticed a couple, but the longer I looked, the more blackheads and enlarged pores I could see. I kept looking at him, and I kept finding other imperfections: He had a few gray hairs, his legs were not as tan as his arms, and his front teeth were not straight . . . and so forth.

I was thrilled, because this little experiment proved my point: Everything and everybody can be improved. The more you look for imperfections, the more you will find them. So, if you are a perfectionist by nature, you won't be ready to settle for anything short of perfect beauty in yourself. Naturally you will be disappointed when you look in the mirror. Your tolerance for even minor appearance flaws might be limited, and even minor flaws may seem huge and obvious, because you will pay more attention to them than would the average person.

In the name of perfection, people lose their jobs and families just because all their time and energy gets gobbled up in appearance improvement rituals. Rick has no friends and has not worked in years, because he is too anxious to tolerate social situations. He feels that people are constantly looking at him. Rick, an absolutely normal-looking Caucasian man, is preoccupied with his skin, which he believes is too pale. He spends several hours per day applying makeup and checking his appearance in the mirror. He also goes to tanning salons regularly and has often burned his skin, because he exposed it to the sun for too long. Rick's wife is considering divorce. She's tired of his appearance obsession, "fed up" with Rick's constant requests for reassurance, and does not understand why he can't work.

Interestingly, people like Rick often use extreme words like looks "ugly" and "awful" when they describe their appearance, but when asked to look at a photo of themselves and rate their appearance on a scale from 0 (*very unattractive*) to 7 (*very attractive*), they rate themselves as 3–4, which, of course, is in the "average" range. It's not that they view themselves as hideous after all; they are just extremely bothered by not reaching their own high appearance standards. One woman who admitted that her friends would probably describe her as average protested, "I just don't want to be mediocre! It is terrible to be mediocre! Nobody will notice me." Apparently, if these people are not absolutely gorgeous—if they manifest anything less than perfection, they must be really ugly.

Is perfectionism an issue for you? On page 32 is a self-test that can help you find out.

Fear of Disapproval

Julia, a 20-year-old college freshman with long black hair and big, dark brown eyes, says she "hates" her looks, despite the fact that most people would consider her appearance well above average, as I do. "It is almost like I see myself through other people's eyes," she explains. "When I walk into a room, I think that everyone is looking at my zits. Then I feel ashamed. I can't relax. My feelings are always on a roller coaster. Whenever I am around others, I feel tense. I worry that they judge the way I look. And it's actually not just about my appearance. When I say something in class, I am really worried that someone might think it was stupid. And when I do something creative, like write something for school, and the professor is not ecstatic about it, I doubt that I will be able to get my degree. Unless people are cheering me all the time, I think they look down on everything I do. I am always afraid that people might somehow find fault with me." Julia demonstrates the reason that many people can't just stop being perfectionists, even when they realize the tendency can be so harmful to them. Many people think their perfectionism is necessary, that it protects them.

If you are very self-conscious about your appearance, you are probably worried that others may find fault with the way you look. You might be concerned that they'll tease you, look down on you, or reject you. Therefore, you do whatever is in your power to improve your appearance. Your fear of disapproval may be the engine for your perfectionism.

How Biological Factors Create Body Image Problems

So far, in this chapter I've discussed mostly external factors, such as culture and psychological theories to explain the development of BDD. However, most psychiatric disorders seem to be at least partially biologically based. Recently some very interesting neurobiological theories for the development of BDD have been proposed.

Is Something Wrong with My Brain?

New imaging technologies allow us to search for abnormalities in the brain. Recently my colleagues, Dr. Scott Rauch and Katharine Phillips, conducted a

Get a Clue: Are You a Perfectionist?

Do any of these statements describe you? If you agree with all or most of them, you might very well be a perfectionist.

You have very high standards. If you cannot do something really well, you feel like you shouldn't do it all.

    Yes or No

If you made a minor mistake at something, you feel like you failed the whole task.

    Yes or No

It is difficult for you to enjoy your accomplishments because they never seem good enough.

    Yes or No

You think that others will not respect you unless you do a perfect job at everything you try.

    Yes or No

You must be excellent at things that matter to you. If you just do an average job, you feel like a second-rate person.

    Yes or No

You spend a lot of time on things that are actually not that important. But you must keep working on them until they are absolutely perfect.

    Yes or No

morphometric resonance imaging study, which provides images of the structure of the brain. They found that scans of the brains of patients with BDD differed in some ways from those of the healthy control participants. Specifically, patients with BDD had a leftward shift in caudate asymmetry, which means that the region of the brain called the *left caudate* was relatively larger than the right caudate. The caudate is involved in regulating movements, thoughts, and feelings. Patients with BDD also had greater total white matter volume than normal controls. These findings of structural brain differences in BDD have to be interpreted with caution given that they were based on only a small sample (eight patients with BDD and eight healthy controls). However, they might indicate that certain brain areas play a role in the development of symptoms related to BDD.

Similar to the results of the neuroimaging study, neuropsychological research that requires patients to use certain brain areas (for example, by drawing a complex figure from memory or recalling long lists of words) also implicates certain brain regions in BDD (for example, the caudate, as well as the orbitofrontal cortex).

Your brain consists of billions of nerve cells or neurons. These nerve cells communicate with the help of brain chemicals that carry messages from one cell to another. Serotonin, one of many chemicals that help transmit information within the brain, plays an important role in regulating your mood and the way you think, your hunger and eating behavior, sleep, aggressive behavior, sexual behavior, and many other bodily functions. It also seems to be important in many psychiatric disorders, such as depression and anxiety disorders. Interestingly, some drugs that distort perception and cause visual illusions (for example, LSD) also affect serotonin. So serotonin might play a role in vision and perception.

As I will describe more in Chapter 10, we know that the medications that help patients with BDD increase the availability of serotonin in the brain. Therefore, it is possible that serotonin plays a role in body image disturbance. Another chemical messenger that may play a role, especially in people with delusional BDD, is dopamine. So, in people with delusional BDD, both serotonin and dopamine may be important.

Further evidence for a potential biological basis of BDD comes from our observations of animals that excessively groom or pick at themselves. Birds may pick at their feathers over and over again, and dogs and cats may compulsively lick their fur, which can result in bald patches and severe skin damage. These animal behaviors look very similar to excessive skin picking and hair combing in BDD, and interestingly enough, several reports indicate that the animals can be treated successfully with medications that affect serotonin (selective serotonin reuptake inhibitors, or SSRIs).

Now, after reading this section, you may think: Since SSRIs help some people with BDD and animals that groom themselves excessively, my problem must have been caused by a serotonin imbalance. This is certainly possible, but there are several problems with this assumption. First, a problem with serotonin does not automatically cause body image disturbance. As you might remember, I said earlier that serotonin might also play a role in depression and various other disorders. So why does one person develop an anxiety disorder, another person develop depression, and still another develop BDD? Well, scientists do not yet know the answers to these questions, but we need to consider that serotonin is not the only chemical messenger in the brain, and different brain chemical systems might be involved in different disorders. For example, dopamine is a messenger that may be relevant for people with delusional thinking. So, in people with delusional BDD, both serotonin and dopamine may be important.

Another issue to consider when wondering whether you might have a chemical imbalance is that although someone might have a good response to an SSRI, this does not necessarily mean that his or her body image problem was caused by not having enough serotonin in the brain. Our brain chemistry changes whenever our mood changes. Therefore, it could actually be the case that your brain has changed as a *result* of having a body image problem. We don't know what came first, the changes in brain chemistry or the changes in mood.

Moreover, it could eventually turn out that a chemical imbalance such as a problem with serotonin provides only the basis to develop a disorder, but our environment determines the specifics of the problem. So, for example, if your family placed a lot of emphasis on good looks, you would be more likely to develop BDD or an eating disorder, but if your parents taught you that you are very vulnerable and the world is a dangerous place, you would be more likely to develop an anxiety disorder.

Did I Inherit My Body Image Problem?

If you have a parent who also struggles with his or her appearance, you might wonder whether you inherited your appearance obsession, and whether you'll pass it on to your kids. Dr. Phillips found that 20% of patients with BDD had at least one first-degree relative with BDD, and that 5.8% of all first-degree relatives had BDD. If we estimate that the prevalence of BDD in the general population is around 1–2%, the rate of BDD in first-degree relatives seems substantially elevated. However, although this research indicates that BDD runs in families, it doesn't necessarily indicate that body image problems are inherited, because we not only share genes with family members but usually also live in the same environment. So if your father is extremely concerned about having smooth skin and you are too, this could be a result of not only learning about the importance of smooth skin from your dad but also something "biological" that was passed on to you. The only way to tease apart environmental and physical factors is through twin and adoption studies, which have not been done in BDD.

Drs. Katharine Phillips and James Kennedy recently examined certain genes they thought likely to be important in BDD. They compared the alleles (forms) of these genes in individuals with and without BDD. Their results showed that people with BDD are more likely to have the short form of the serotonin transporter region gene. This gene codes for something called the *serotonin transporter*, which is the system that recycles serotonin from the spaces between the brain nerve cells. Serotonin reuptake inhibitor (SRI) medications target the serotonin transporter. The results by Drs. Kennedy and Phillips suggest that the short allele of this gene may increase the risk for the development of BDD.

Drs. Phillips and Kennedy also found that one form of the GABA (a neurotransmitter that inhibits nerve activity) gene is associated with BDD. This truly groundbreaking work is the first genetics study in BDD. However, it is important to point out that BDD most likely involves several different genes, which interact with each other and the environmental factors described earlier. It's quite possible that whereas you have inherited from one of your parents a biological vulnerability to some kind of psychiatric problem, the actual problem may have been triggered by some kind of external factor, such as teasing or other environmental circumstances.

The Mind as a Filter

The groundwork for your excessive appearance concerns could have been laid down in your childhood your parents' comments, by the types of toys you played with and the commercial and cultural messages you received, and by personality traits that you developed, such as perfectionism and fear of disapproval. Biological factors, such as your brain chemicals and your genes, might also affect your body image. All of these factors might influence how you interpret your looks and the world around you. Your mind serves as a filter that actually reinforces your worst fears and most dangerous assumptions about your looks.

If you are like most people with appearance concerns, you may believe that the first thing others notice about you is your flaw, that other people are staring at you, that any negative interaction with others is a response to your defect. And no matter how often your family members and friends try to provide you with other explanations, you don't believe them. Why not?

Because your mind colors what you attend to and remember in any situation, once you have a certain belief, you easily notice and recognize things that confirm this belief, and you are more likely to ignore or forget anything that contradicts it. It is as if you have a filter in front of your eyes. So, for example, if you hold the belief "I am ugly," anything that fits the belief that you are unattractive will go right through the filter and into your head. But if something does not agree with the belief "I am ugly," you either won't notice it or you will alter it in some way, so that it eventually agrees with the belief. Let's say someone pays you a compliment. Do you believe this person was really trying to say that you look good? Or do you think something like: "He just says this because he knows how much I struggle with my appearance!" Or someone says, "You look really nice today!" Do you immediately think, "Is she trying to tell me that I look bad on other days?"

Like many people with a negative body image, you probably picked up various beliefs about looking unattractive or having to look perfect as a child, and these are the filters through which all your later perceptions have to pass before being processed by your mind. It's not your fault that you acquired those beliefs when young, but it is your challenge as an adult to think these assumptions through. The good news is that since beliefs are learned, you can unlearn them if they turn out to be unhelpful or faulty.

How does the filter operate when you look in the mirror? For a long time, body image researchers discussed the following question: Is there a sensory disturbance that might contribute to a poor body image? That is, do the eyes send a different signal to the brain while checking the mirror? Or is the poor body image related mostly to the person's attitudes toward his or her own body?

What Do You See?

It's possible that disturbed serotonin levels in the brain lead to faulty perception or to faulty interpretation of visual images. Research on patients with BDD has yet to be done. Most researchers who work with eating disorders believe that perception can in fact be altered in these patients, but not because their senses work differently. Rather, they believe that people with BDD and negative body image perceive themselves, and those with whom they compare themselves, differently than do other people mostly because of emotional and thinking processes. In other words, your visual system probably works just fine, but your mind interprets what you see in a negative way. Again, the filter is at work.

What you see when you look in the mirror becomes a matter of selective attention: You see only whatever defect bothers you and pretty much ignore the rest of your reflection. We see this selective attention quite often in our patients with BDD, and it also matches some results we obtained with the Rey–Osterrieth Complex Figure Test. When drawing this complex figure from memory, participants with BDD tended to focus on details rather than larger, organizational design features. They had trouble seeing the "big picture," which resulted in memory deficits. Overfocusing on details is likely related to the development and maintenance of BDD's clinical features. Indeed, it appears that people with BDD focus on certain aspects of their body, ignoring global aspects of appearance, and thereby distort self-perception.

What are you focusing on when you look in the mirror? Do you pay attention to the features you like? Or do you focus only on whatever bothers you?

Looking only at your flaws could lead to a perceptual distortion that makes your defect appear very noticeable. At the same time, if you believe you are ugly, your filter will screen out your acceptable features. This way, even a pore or minor scar might seem enormous to you. It is likely that the all the attention you pay to your minor flaws might contribute to or maintain the problem you have with your body image.

Believing Is Seeing . . . and, in Turn, Behaving

One important way that your beliefs work is by directly influencing your behavior. If you grew up in a family with a huge focus on appearance, you might have learned a belief along the lines of "My physical appearance is a sign of my inner worth" or "My appearance has to be perfect." Now you know that such a belief will probably cause you to pay a lot of attention to your looks and to be extremely concerned about every wrinkle, pimple, or lost hair. But it will also, in turn, influence how you feel and behave.

When Gina was 11, her father told her, "It's not gonna be easy to find you a husband. You better work hard in school, because you'll never be beautiful." For all the reasons we believe everything our parents tell us, Gina believed she would never be beautiful. And her mind filtered out any evidence that, in fact, she was perfectly nice looking, so by the time she was a young adult, she felt very ashamed about her looks. To feel better, she got herself into a self-improvement frenzy. She got facial implants and had liposuction. But no matter what kind of surgery she had, Gina was never satisfied with the outcome. Her appearance concerns also led her to feel quite anxious in social situations, and she avoided them whenever she could. Since Gina rarely socialized, she never got to date, which only served to reinforce her beliefs that she was unlovable and defective.

Triggering Events

So far we've discussed what might cause your appearance concerns, and the appearance rituals and avoidance behaviors that maintain them. However, body image theories should also account for why BDD begins when it does. Sometimes appearance concerns get triggered by a teasing incident or a specific comment, as with Gina or Yolanda. At other times, they follow a negative life event, such as a breakup of a romantic relationship or getting laid off at work. At times, BDD seems to respond to more general stressors, like starting a new job, moving to another city, or having marital or occupational problems. Most of the time BDD begins in adolescence, which makes you wonder to what degree the sudden changes in appearance that occur at this time trigger body image problems.

Fear of Physical Change at Critical Points in the Lifespan

We all know that there are certain times in our lives when we feel particularly vulnerable to criticism, when our bodies (and minds) are changing, and we fear that our new selves won't be considered worthy and acceptable. Adolescence is primary among those transitions and, not surprisingly, it's the typical age of onset for BDD. Obviously, the physical changes of adolescence are dramatic. Breasts may develop excessively, skin may break out, and hair may grow in unwanted areas. Adolescents tend be more interested in appearance, and if they look different from their friends, they might feel self-conscious and be teased by peers. Most adolescents have issues with their appearance, but BDD is much more severe than the typical appearance concerns of adolescence.

Adolescents with BDD are severely distressed; often their schoolwork suffers, and they may avoid going to social events and withdraw from friends or family. Wayne, a 16-year-old honor student in a prestigious high school, is smart and an excellent athlete. His parents brought him in to treatment because they were concerned about his shyness. "Wayne really doesn't have any friends. When someone invites him, he makes up excuses. He shows up in class at the last minute, so he doesn't have to talk to anyone. His skin has been breaking out a little in the past few years, which has bothered him a lot. Lots of kids have acne that's much worse, though, and they still go out and make friends. And recently he started making these requests for plastic surgery. He wants to have his nose fixed."

Wayne tells me that when people look at his face, he's worried that they are thinking about his nose or his pimples. Although he has always been shy in social situations, since he started having these nose concerns, he does not feel like socializing at all. When I asked Wayne why he started being so concerned about his appearance, he told me: "Everyone in my class is worried about how they look. Looking good is important for all kids my age. And there are several kids in my school who had surgery. I think my problems are worse than theirs, but it's the same basic issue."

Do body image concerns start or get worse when people get older because people cannot handle the effects of aging? I've never seen a patient whose BDD started in old age and, to my knowledge, this question hasn't been researched. But many people who have had various body image problems over the course of their lives also experience major difficulties with the signs of aging. Katinka is a tall, amazingly beautiful woman in her early 30s. She used to work as a model and had multiple plastic surgeries, which she told me is actually quite common in her profession. When her first tiny wrinkles appeared in her late 20s, she panicked. Although she sometimes realized that her looks were way above average, she usually told me, "I look old and ugly!" During those times, she was afraid she would no longer be special to her husband. "What's left if I don't have my looks? That's all I have going for myself. Why would he want to stay with me?" These statements were quite surprising for someone who actually was very intelligent, educated, and just a great person with whom to talk. To deal with her fears of aging, Katinka frequently got Botox injections and underwent multiple chemical peels. She also got herself into an exercise frenzy. No matter what she did, she was not satisfied with her appearance. Only after several months of treatment was she able to stop the negative thoughts about her looks and her excessive appearance rituals.

Understanding Your Body Image: How Do the Puzzle Pieces Fit Together?

In summary, there is a wide range of possible triggers for severe body image concerns, including stress, negative comments, and physical changes related to adolescence and, less frequently, aging. Although researchers have started to do a lot of research on body image, we do not yet know whether biological or environmental influences are more important in causing body image disturbances. As illustrated in the diagram below, cultural influences, the messages you got from your family and peers, certain personality styles, and disturbed brain chemistry might all have contributed to the problems you have with accepting your looks. Not only does your problem probably have multiple sources, but it is also likely that the different factors interact in a complex pattern.

What Causes Body Image Concerns?

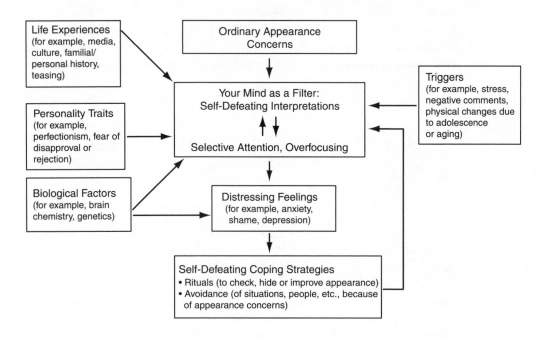

Everyone has some minor flaws in appearance and occasionally thinks about them. What separates you from people with a good body image is not that you have minor flaws in appearance but how you react to them. Whereas many people can just disregard their minor appearance flaws, people with a problematic body image focus on them and consider them important. Such an intense and negative evaluation of flaws might be influenced by perfectionistic beliefs about appearance or by assumptions that these flaws reveal something bad about the person's character. If you are very fearful of negative evaluation by others, you are also more likely to develop appearance concerns.

Your beliefs about your appearance might have developed because of a biological vulnerability, family and cultural values, or childhood experiences. Other factors, such as stress, certain negative comments, and current mood, may also play a role in the way you react to an appearance flaw, as the diagram shows. If you notice an imperfection in your appearance, you'll have negative feelings such as anxiety, sadness, shame, or disgust. Because nobody likes to feel bad, you'll think of something to stop or avoid these feelings.

For example, you avoid or escape from situations that trigger them. Another way of dealing with the unpleasant feeling is to engage in one of your beauty rituals (for example, mirror checking, reassurance seeking, exercising). Avoidance behavior, hiding the defect, or checking may relieve the anxiety or shame for a little while. Therefore, you may find yourself wanting to resort to these measures over and over again. In the long term, however, they are the engine that maintains your negative beliefs, because every time you avoid or ritualize you lose an opportunity to learn that things would have turned out OK if you had just faced the situation without compulsions.

In the next chapters, you'll learn more about how your thoughts influence your feelings and actions. More important, I'll also show you what you can do to change your negative thinking, as well as your appearance rituals and avoidance behavior, which will lead to greater self-acceptance and enhanced confidence.

Chapter 3

Thinking about Change

What if I said that you could solve the problem that brought you to this book by changing the way you think?

Your instinctive reaction might be "I don't have a problem with my thinking. My problem is the way I look!" Or it might be "Great! I might actually learn how to deal with these awful thoughts and these time-wasting habits." Or it might be anything in between. Whatever your reaction, your feelings will follow directly from your thoughts.

If you had the first reaction, you might feel disappointed to hear that we'll work on changing your thinking. You might even feel angry, because I may have reminded you of something that someone in your family has told you before. You might even put the book down.

If you had the second reaction, you might feel a little excited, eager to read on.

In either case, you might say this book had caused you to feel the way you feel. But how could exactly the same book evoke two widely different feelings? Because it's not the book itself that caused you to have certain feelings or perform certain actions; it's how you *think* about the book.

Your feelings are directly linked to and influenced by your thoughts. If you feel anxious or inadequate in social situations, you may think this is because you are not attractive enough to feel satisfied or self-confident. If you have beliefs such as "My life would be so much better if I were more attractive," or "I have to look perfect," or "I'm so ugly," you will notice an imperfection in your appearance much more than the average person does, and it will seem huge and obvious to you. You will also have negative feelings such as anxiety, sadness, shame, or even disgust in response to your imperfections. Because nobody likes to feel bad, you'll come up with a way to stop or avoid these feelings, and quite possibly stay away from situations that trigger them when you can and escape posthaste when you can't. Another way of dealing with the unpleasant feelings is to perform one of your beauty rituals, whether it's mirror checking, reassurance seeking, or exercising. All of these behaviors—avoiding triggering situations, hiding your "defects," and checking on your appearance—may relieve the anxiety or shame for a little while. This will probably convince you to resort to these behaviors over and over again. The way you think about your appearance obviously determines how you feel and react in various situations.

Changing the way you think about your appearance, so that you can gradually decrease problematic behaviors and start spending your time on more rewarding pursuits, is what this program is all about. The name for this approach is *cognitive-behavioral therapy* (CBT), a type of treatment that has been effective in helping people eliminate or improve a lot of other problems, from anxiety and depression to excessive drinking and eating disorders. In the case of appearance concerns, there are a number of possible routes to improvement, including medications (described in Chapter 10) and CBT. CBT for BDD has proven to be highly effective. No self-help outcome data were available when this book was published, but for a 12-session individual outpatient treatment, you can expect an average of about 47–51% decrease in symptoms. The lower figure is from my own ongoing, individual treatment trial, which includes patients with very severe BDD; the higher number is from a published trial by David Veale that included patients with milder BDD.

CBT actually encompasses several different treatment techniques. The cognitive part of the treatment focuses on cognitions—your thoughts, perceptions, and beliefs. Your thoughts run through your mind all day long and have a profound impact on how you feel. If you constantly feel anxious or upset, or depressed or frustrated about how you look, it could be because of certain thoughts that are always simmering in your brain. One of the goals of CBT is to evaluate and, if necessary, modify how you think. You may find this hard to believe right now, but your thoughts, perceptions, and beliefs about your appearance may not be entirely accurate. Maybe they are exaggerated or in some other way not based in reality. CBT can teach you how to recognize what is faulty or unhelpful about your thinking and change it.

The behavioral aspect of CBT focuses on the mirror checking, skin picking, avoidance of social situations, and other ways you act in response to the uncomfortable feelings caused by thoughts about your appearance. The goal is to decrease these behaviors and to develop healthier ones in their place.

Thinking about Change: A Cost–Benefit Analysis

This brief description of CBT and my claim that it can help you solve the problem that led you to this book by helping you change the way you think are probably not enough to convince you to try this program right now. The fact that you *are* reading this book, of course, indicates that you believe something about your life isn't what it could be. At the very least you want to understand better what's happening to you and whether there is anything you can and should do differently. Chapters 1 and 2 should have started to answer those questions, and maybe you're more certain than you used to be that there's reason to think about change. But there may very well be a nagging voice at the back of your head (or even up front) that still says that everything would be just fine if only you could fix that bump in your nose, or try dermabrasion one more time, or get just a little more ripped, or find the perfect hairstyle once and for all.

Should you keep trying to improve your appearance, then, or should you try something else? If you were at work, there's a good chance that your company would approach a question like that by performing a cost–benefit analysis. What would you stand to gain from either approach, and how much would it cost?

What Is Your Poor Body Image Costing You?

Different people are affected by their appearance concerns in different ways. Heidi was really disturbed about the fact that her problem limited her activities: "You know, it's hard to enjoy the beach if you're preoccupied with how your breasts are sagging and your freckles are showing. So I just don't want to go there anymore!" Carlos was mostly worried about the negative impact his problems had on his social life: "It's difficult to ask someone for a date when I'm worried that the girls are disgusted with my nose and with the hair on my body. I don't even try to ask girls out, because I don't want to put anyone in an awkward situation." Marisa mentioned the emotional consequences: "I'm so short, my hair is so red, my skin is so white, and then I have this scar on my cheek. I feel like an ugly duckling, and I often wonder if people feel sorry for me. When they look at me they probably think: 'This poor little thing. Look how pale and sick she is.' I have no self-esteem and feel ashamed all the time."

If you've struggled with poor body image for quite some time, you've probably adjusted your life to accommodate your problem. Maybe you don't even register all of the consequences of poor body image as costs, because they are "just the way things are." The exercise on pages 44–45 will help you identify the true costs of your body image issues.

How many negative consequences did you check off? Probably more than you would have expected. Are the problems caused by your appearance concerns pervasive? Does that surprise you?

Many people with body image problems are not aware of the huge toll their problem has taken on their life. They know they have accommodated their problem somehow, but they have never taken a good look at the disadvantages

Assessing the Cost of Appearance Concerns

Check each item that applies to you. Try to take some time to think, or go through the list more than once. Body image problems can have mental, emotional, social, financial, and practical consequences, so be sure to consider each possibility seriously.

- ❏ Dissatisfaction
- ❏ Shame/embarrassment
- ❏ Guilt
- ❏ Anxiety
- ❏ Concern that your children will become preoccupied with appearance
- ❏ Loneliness/isolation
- ❏ Decreased self-esteem
- ❏ Jealousy of better-looking people
- ❏ Self-hate
- ❏ Disgust
- ❏ Anger
- ❏ Fear of rejection or abandonment
- ❏ Fear of being ridiculed
- ❏ Avoidance of intimate relationships
- ❏ Arguments over beauty rituals or cost of beauty products
- ❏ Stress on relationship due to avoidance behaviors or comparing
- ❏ Making excuses or lying about the problem
- ❏ Not going to school/work because of appearance concerns
- ❏ Being late for school/work because of beauty rituals
- ❏ Avoidance of body-focused activities (for example, swimming, gym)
- ❏ Refusing overnight trips because they limit privacy
- ❏ Avoiding people of the opposite sex
- ❏ Avoidance of social activities that others consider to be fun (for example, parties, eating out)
- ❏ Avoidance of revealing clothes

(continued)

Assessing the Cost of Appearance Concerns *(continued)*

- ❏ Avoidance of getting your picture taken

- ❏ Avoidance of mirrors

- ❏ Avoidance of being seen from certain angles

- ❏ Avoidance of certain task (for example, sitting near a window or under bright lights)

- ❏ Time for rituals (for example, mirror checking, comparing, shopping, appearance fixing, beauty and doctors appointments, recovery from surgery)

- ❏ Scarring as result of surgery, or self-surgery

- ❏ Skin damage (for example, result of picking, sunburns, tanning)

- ❏ Scabs or scarring as result of skin picking

- ❏ Pain as result of surgery

- ❏ Harm to muscles and joints due to excessive exercise

- ❏ Accidents (due to mirror checking)

- ❏ Alcohol and drug use to cope with preoccupation

- ❏ Cost of beauty products to hide or improve aspects of appearance (for example, makeup, hair products, soaps, skin cream)

- ❏ Cost of spas (for example, hairdressers, estheticians)

- ❏ Cost of dental, surgical, or dermatological treatments

- ❏ Cost of psychiatric treatments

- ❏ Cost of hats and clothing

- ❏ Others:

_____

_____

_____

of being obsessed with their appearance. Now that you have seen this list, how would you answer the following questions?

Do you want to change?

Do you want to stop being so obsessed with your looks?

Do you want to stop comparing?

Are you tired of being scared of mirrors?

If your answer is "yes" to any of these questions, know that it is certainly possible to change. It is possible to be happy and confident around others and in front of the mirror. Maybe you feel that a change requires more willpower or self-discipline than you've been able to muster. To enhance your motivation to try to change, think about the effect your body image problem might

> "I thought I looked really disgusting. I still don't think that I look like Superman, but I can accept myself now!"
>
> —*Vincent, age 34*

have had on your life. Understand, though, that your willingness to change might waver as you work your way through the program in this book, so refer back to this list from time to time. This might help sustain your motivation. Also understand that one of the distinct advantages of CBT is that it reinforces itself as you go along. You may need motivation to get started and also to get over any sizable humps, but for the most part, the treatment itself will provide ongoing motivation. That's because it works. CBT can give you major and lasting improvements in the way you feel, see yourself, and interact with others, and it can increase your productivity and accomplishments. CBT is effective, works fast, is simple in theory, is easy to learn, and, unlike many medications, does not have any physical side effects. In the last few years, researchers (myself included) in the United States, and some in the United Kingdom, have successfully developed and tested CBT for BDD. These studies have shown

> "I'm so much happier now. I used to spend so much time at home, hiding. . . . Now I feel free. I have a really good life!"
>
> —*Louisa, age 49*

consistently that programs similar to the one described in this book help people with body image problems.

How does this apply to you? Now that you know what your appearance concerns are costing you, you should look at the benefits of change.

What Benefits Can You Expect from Change?

If you were to get control over your appearance obsession, what would be different? Make a list of any positive consequences you can think of. The list of negative consequences that you prepared earlier might help you with this exercise. Just pick the negative consequences that bother you most and list the corresponding positive change.

The following questions might also be useful.

If I improved my body image . . .

- Would this have an impact on my self-esteem?
- Would I feel better?
- Would it improve the quality of my life? If so, how?
- Would it improve the quality of my relationships with others?
- Would it improve my performance at school or work?
- Would I have more time or money for things I'd actually enjoy?
- Would it improve my health?

Golda was sad about the way she felt about herself. "I just don't like myself. I have very little self-respect, and that's because I think I am not pretty. I hate the zits and wrinkles on my face. And then I have this flabby stomach.. ..I'm addicted to dermabrasions. And I keep buying all kinds of things to smear on my face—makeup, face creams, facials, you name it. And the amount of time I spend in the gym—it's just crazy. Sometimes I go to the gym instead of meeting friends. It just takes too much time, and it's really not fun. . . . And despite all of this, I still don't feel better about the way I look. I'm often late for things because I'm busy picking my skin or putting on makeup. Whenever my friends ask me to go camping, I have to make up excuses, because I don't want them to know how long it takes me to get ready. And I don't really want anyone to see me without makeup anyway. I also don't like it when my boyfriend touches my face, and I'm really self-conscious about my stomach. . . . I'm tired of this. I just want to enjoy my life and not think about this stuff all the time."

Her list of the advantages of change looked like this:

1. Improved self-esteem. I'll respect myself. I will feel better about my body.
2. Less anxiety when someone looks at me.
3. I'll be able to get to my classes on time.
4. I'll be able to go to the beach and parties and enjoy it.
5. I'll be able to think of other things besides appearance.
6. I'll be able to go camping with friends.
7. More energy to build relationships, paint, and write.
8. I can save money to travel to Europe.
9. I'll be able to have other people come close to my face.
10. I'll be able to let others touch my face.

At the end of the program Golda told me, "I used this list as a motivator. I actually taped it on my fridge, and when the going got tough, I looked at it.

It was really helpful, especially during times when I was discouraged or afraid to start a new exercise. It's funny, now that I'm done with the program, I've noticed even more advantages, things that I couldn't even imagine when I first started. Like doing so much better in school because I can concentrate on my work now, and making new friends because I'm more outgoing."

"I am so proud that I completed this program. It was difficult to admit that I have a problem, but I just could not go on. Now I feel normal again. Like I did before I got so obsessed with my skin. It only takes me 25 minutes to get ready in the morning, and I have not been to a dermatologist in months. Even my husband noticed that I am so much happier and less irritable now!"

—Hilda, age 29

Once you've prepared your own list of advantages, the next step is to imagine how good it would feel for you to graduate from this program and enjoy all of the benefits you listed. Fantasize about how much you would like getting control over your appearance obsession. Imagine all the different things you could enjoy that you are avoiding or enduring with anxiety now. Think about all the money and time you would save—and how you would spend it. Picture yourself happier and more self-confident.

People are often amazed at how much better they feel once they've improved their body image. But you haven't gotten there yet, so perhaps you're still skeptical. Let's return to hard data.

How Much Will It Cost to Change?

It wouldn't be a very fair analysis if you considered only the costs of not changing and the benefits of changing. You also have to consider potential reasons not to change.

• **Trying to change means taking a risk.** Sometimes people have asked me: "What if at the end it turns out that I haven't improved at all? I'll feel like such a failure." The techniques described in the program are very powerful and have been proven to work in research on patients undergoing individual or group treatment. So you have every reason to expect to get better. You can't expect your appearance obsessions to improve if you keep using your old strategies. If they were effective, they would have worked by now. In the unlikely event that this book does not help you, there are many other options you can pursue. But if you don't try this program, you will never know whether it could have worked for you. The vast majority of people that I've helped work on their body image problems have felt that the risk of failure or wasted time associated with CBT is worthwhile, and very few have dropped out of individual treatment.

- **Giving up appearance rituals might mean looking even worse.** You might also be worried about the implications of behavior changes that this program requires. Carina was concerned about what would happen if she decreased her efforts to improve her appearance. "What will happen to my skin? I'm really afraid to stop going to dermatologists. Am I not supposed to have any plastic surgery at all? And what about facial creams? Can I use them at least? I'm afraid that I'll look really ugly at the end of this program. I'll probably get zits and wrinkles. I can't afford to let myself go like this!" Many people with appearance concerns are very afraid to make behavioral changes. Some people are worried that their appearance fears might be confirmed and that their appearance will somehow get out of control. At the beginning of CBT I only ask people to delay any major appearance changes such as plastic surgery, hair transplants, and so forth. Later I ask that they gradually reduce less drastic appearance rituals, such as excessive makeup application, mirror checking, and skin picking. The simple truth is that it would be best for you to learn to live with an occasional imperfection. Even if you have spent huge amounts of time battling pimples or wrinkles, by now you may have realized that once in a while you will get one anyway. The battle for perfection and going against your biology is futile. Therefore, I recommend that you try to accept your appearance imperfections for now and then reevaluate your progress in 2 months. At that point, you can decide whether you still feel the need for surgery or other time-consuming beauty rituals.

- **Letting go of appearance rituals might mean *feeling* worse.** People often tell me that they are very afraid to let go of their appearance rituals, because the rituals temporarily make them feel better. While it's true that your discomfort or anxiety will probably increase when you first try to cut down on your beauty rituals, most likely your discomfort will be much lower than you initially expect. Usually people tell me that the anxiety they feel when they worry about changing their behavior is much worse than any anxiety that results from changing the behavior itself. Even if your anxiety rises initially, you can be assured that this is only temporary. If you keep resisting your beauty rituals, your anxiety will automatically decrease on its own. Inga used to put a lot of makeup on her face to camouflage her freckles. "When I thought about going to a shopping mall without makeup, the anxiety mounted to a fairly high level right away. But when I actually did it, it was not so bad at all. The first 5 minutes were kind of tough, but then the anxiety really diminished over the next 15 or 20 minutes."

You may feel a little anxious when you first change your behavior, but you will certainly feel a great sense of accomplishment after each step of the program is completed. That's how CBT provides the ongoing motivation I mentioned earlier. Also, be assured that my goal is only to challenge you with this program, not to overwhelm you! We'll proceed in a gradual manner, and you'll overcome your problems by first changing your self-defeating thoughts and then setting realistic goals and creating exercises for yourself. We'll rank your exercises from easy to difficult, and you'll start with the easier ones. Therefore, your anxiety will always be tolerable, and your chances of success will be maximized.

Here's how this gradual approach worked for one of my patients. Tobias, a geneticist, was very intelligent but highly anxious. He felt uncomfortable in most social situations because he thought his nose was too long. He was anxious around his colleagues, neighbors, and just about everyone except his wife and two sons. He dreaded eye contact and mostly went to "safe" places, where he felt like his appearance was not noticed. Giving a presentation during the grand rounds in his department was his top treatment goal. The thought of having everyone look at him was incredibly scary, but avoiding research presentations was holding him back at his career. Rather than starting at the top of his list, Tobias began with situations that were only mildly anxiety provoking, such as making eye contact with the salesperson in the local grocery store. When he tried this, his anxiety initially rose a little. But Tobias calmed down quickly, because he realized that rather than staring at his nose, as he had predicted, people were actually quite friendly.

After he had mastered several of these initial exercises successfully, Tobias was ready to take on more challenging tasks. He decided that he wanted to try sitting right next to one of his female colleagues in a research meeting. This was quite difficult, because he was concerned that she could see his profile and would be appalled by his long nose. At the beginning of his CBT program, this goal would have felt completely out of reach. But by now he was more confident. Tobias had learned to manage his thoughts (with the techniques described in Chapter 4), and he also had plenty of experience with exposing himself to less anxiety-provoking situations. So he went ahead and sat right next to his attractive colleague, and to make things even more challenging, four other people were also attending the meeting. People could actually see his face from all angles! They had a productive meeting, discussing new ideas for future projects. Nobody stared at his nose, looked appalled, or made a demeaning comment about his appearance. In fact, people seemed very pleased with his presence and his contributions to the topics under discussion. His anxiety peaked initially whenever somebody looked at him directly, but this improved quickly, and by the end of the meeting, Tobias felt pretty good about being been able to do this exercise.

Tobias completed his treatment about 3 years ago and has given grand rounds and many talks at national and international conferences since. "I feel so much more confident," he says, "and so much happier, because I can do the things I always wanted to do. Sometimes it was hard to do the exercises, but it was definitely worth it."

 • **Trying to change will take a lot of time and effort.** This may be true. CBT requires commitment and time. But will it take more time than you now spend on assuaging your appearance concerns? Look back at your list of the costs of having a poor body image. How much of your time each day is spent dealing with appearance concerns, whether it's thinking about your looks, time spent on beauty rituals, or time spent working late because worrying about your looks has robbed you of the concentration you need to get your work done during normal working hours? Let's assume that you spend about 2 hours per day thinking about your appearance or doing rituals to improve, hide, or check your looks. This is about twice as much time as you would have to invest per day in this self-help program, which would last only about 12 weeks (depending on the severity of your problem, the duration of this program could be shorter or longer).

The numbers are even more impressive if you consider how much time your body image problems cost you in the long run. If you have mild problems, it would be about 60 hours per month, or 720 hours per year, or 43,200 hours over your lifetime (if we assume that you live until you are 77 years old and your appearance preoccupation started when you were 17). Of course, if your body image problem is moderate or severe, those numbers would be even higher. In any event, the number is huge if you consider that the active phase of our CBT self-help program will require only about 84 hours or so (thereafter you will still need to practice, but you'll soon reduce your sessions to about once a month, once a season, or once a year).

If you're still tempted to persist with your old appearance improvement strategies rather than try CBT and change, add up the other costs of trying to change: Risk of failure is low, you don't need to stop grooming yourself or attending to your appearance altogether or all at once; any anxiety you feel from giving up appearance rituals will be short-lived, and you'll probably spend less time and effort on CBT than you do now on trying to improve your appearance or avoid situations that make you worry about your appearance.

I think any good businessperson would say that the cost–benefit analysis gives a message that's loud and clear: Trying to change via CBT leaves you with much to gain and little to lose. This isn't business, though, is it? It's your life, your well-being, your happiness and contentment. We're not talking about a pragmatic matter of tossing out one marketing strategy in favor of another, but about giving up familiar ways of thinking and acting that have become a way of life.

All I can ask you is this: Is it a way of life that you're as comfortable with now as you were in the past? Your reading this book says it's not. When you think about change, think carefully about how well your old strategy worked. Keep reminding yourself of the exercise Assessing the Cost of Appearance Concerns that helped you identify the psychological and physical consequences of your appearance obsessions. Use the benefits you stand to gain from change as a mantra to keep you focused. And remember that, as treatments go, CBT just may be the best bargain you can find.

Who Should Not Use This Program?

You can use this program whether you are male or female, young or old, have mild or severe appearance concerns, and whether you are working on it alone or with a friend, family member, or therapist. However, self-help alone is not enough if

- You are feeling very depressed or suicidal.
- You have problems with alcohol or drugs.
- You have physical problems as a result of your appearance concerns (e.g., due to excessive exercise, dieting, and surgeries).

In any of these cases, you may be able to use this program, but you should also immediately look for a qualified mental health service provider. I provide some resources to help you find a clinician at the end of this book.

Getting the Most Out of the Program

There's a very good reason for weighing the costs and benefits to increase your motivation for starting the program that follows in this book: Your success will depend directly on how *actively* you get involved in this program. I can't emphasize this enough. You can get control over your problem if you practice the exercises provided—not just once or twice, but over and over again. The more you practice, the more you will improve.

Here are a few more tips for success.

One Step at a Time

Your self-help program consists of a number of different components, and it's a good idea to read the chapters in the order in which they are presented in this book. In Chapters 1 and 2, you learned about the nature of body image problems and their causes. In this chapter, you are preparing to get started with the program. Next, I will show you how to control your body image concerns by setting goals for yourself and managing your negative thoughts, reversing patterns of avoidance, and decreasing beauty rituals. Then I provide you with tips about protecting yourself from relapse after you have successfully completed this program. Finally, I offer information about medication treatment, as well as additional resources, including further reading, interesting websites, and guidance on how you can find a clinician.

This is the order in which we teach the different components in CBT in our

> "CBT has helped me a lot. I am not stuck in the mirror anymore, and I rarely pick my skin. I am so much more confident around my friends."
>
> —*Sol, age 24*

"I often think back to skills I have learned in CBT. I behave completely differently, and I think my kids like me better, too. I can accept compliments now and don't ask my husband for reassurance all the time. And I don't waste all this time and money on going to the spa!"

—Dina, age 42

clinic. You will also see that later chapters build on previous ones. Reading the book chapter by chapter, rather than jumping around, will help you stay focused.

You also need to be realistic about what you can do. Add new exercises only after you've mastered the earlier ones.

Most likely, some of the chapters and components of the program will not be as relevant to you as others. Keep in mind that this book is written for everyone who has a body image problem. You might be extremely concerned about your appearance or just a little. You might have unrealistic appearance standards, or you might think you are completely ugly. You might have a mild actual defect in appearance or none at all. You might avoid many situations or none. You might have many rituals or hardly any. Usually it should be pretty clear which sections apply to you. The assessment sections in Chapter 4 will also help you determine which aspects of the program you need to emphasize.

In addition, always remember to take your time. There is no need to rush through the program; just keep trying to make steady progress. Most likely, it will take you a minimum of 12 weeks to complete the program. Sometimes it will be helpful to spend extra time on a section if you feel there is more you could learn.

Review What You've Learned

It's a good idea occasionally to review what you've learned. For example, you could spend about 20 minutes a week revisiting material you've already covered. Especially if you have a setback, you might benefit from reviewing the materials. Also, be sure to monitor your progress. If you're moving ahead, just carry on. However, if you feel that you're stuck, it may be useful to go back and reread the sections that describe the exercises that are difficult for you. If you get stuck for extended periods of time, you may want to consider getting a helper or seeking professional help.

Consider Getting a Helper

Even if you understand the strategies I describe in this book, it may sometimes be challenging to apply them. That's when an encouraging friend or family member can be really useful. If you decide to work with a helper, choose someone you trust and encourage him or her to read this book. Of course, you could also work with a therapist, who could supervise your use of the program.

A Proper Send-Off from Those Who Have Gone Before

A few years ago, several patients who participated in a BDD group run by my colleague Dr. Michael Otto decided to write a message to other people with body image concerns. Here is what they have to say to you:

We have been where you are now, and we want you to know:

We care about you.

You are not alone. Other people have the same problem.

We are glad you are thinking about change.

Be angry at the problem, not at yourself.

Drop the shame. The feelings that you have are not your fault.

Stop criticizing yourself. You are struggling with a problem; treat yourself well.

Pay attention to the things that you enjoy, not your skin, hair, and so forth.

It is the inside that needs your attention, not the outside.

Comparing yourself to others is a waste of time. It is not a competition; it is about enjoying your life.

Don't isolate yourself.

Give yourself credit for the smallest effort.

Try to live in the present. It's all about creating pleasure and meaning in life, not past regrets.

You can't wait to feel good to do something. Sometimes you change how you feel by changing what you do.

It is a progression: Listen, learn, and change your life.

Chapter 4

Understanding
Your Problems
and Planning Solutions

In the previous chapter, we talked about the general goals of this program. You learned that this program helps you change the way you think about your appearance. This will lay the groundwork for gradually reducing problematic behaviors and starting to spend your time on more rewarding things in life. It's normal to have a few doubts about giving up old behaviors and trying new ones. That's why I've encouraged you to weigh the cost of a poor body image against the potential benefits of change. You can now move on to the next step, which involves assessing your behavior and setting goals. But don't forget: If at any point you lose your motivation to continue, you might want to reread Chapter 3.

In this chapter, you'll assess what kind of problems you have and how severe they are. This will help you plan your treatment well. You'll start by assessing your satisfaction with different body parts, then you'll move on to identifying difficult thoughts, stressful situations, and ritualistic behaviors. Most likely, all tests will be relevant for you. There are some people, though, who have only very few or no beauty rituals. That's sometimes because they simply avoid everything that makes them uncomfortable. On the other hand, less frequently, I've also seen people who had hardly any avoidance behavior and just endured difficult situations by preparing with beauty rituals beforehand. Functionally, avoidance behaviors and rituals are the same; they're done to keep your discomfort under control. Unfortunately, the same avoidance behaviors and rituals prevent you from learning to face what you fear—and, more important, they keep you from finding out that things just turn out OK if you face your fears. I'll give you instructions for using the program if you have both rituals and avoidance behaviors, or just one of the two.

The tests on pages 57 and 59–62 will help you identify which areas are hard for you and need work. Once you're done taking the tests, you'll interpret your results. Knowing where you stand right now will help you decide what to focus on in this program and set your long-term goals. Over the course of your program, you'll come back to this section to retake these tests. This will help you evaluate the gains you've made. Because you'll be taking these tests more than once, I recommend that you photocopy the following tests before you fill them out.

Assess Yourself

Assessing Your Satisfaction with Different Body Parts

This first body image test evaluates how much you like or dislike specific features of your body. If some important aspect of your body is not listed, simply add it to the bottom and rate your level of satisfaction with it. Please go ahead and rate your satisfaction with different aspects of your body now.

If you have many features you dislike very much or mostly dislike, your score might be a very high negative number (e.g., over –15), but I've seen patients who had a score of only –3 or –6 on this test and still suffered very much. In any event, if you have a negative score, you beat yourself up for the way you look. The dissatisfaction with your body image likely affects your self-esteem, and it's definitely worthwhile to work on it.

If your score is around 0, you're pretty neutral toward the way you look. You're not terribly dissatisfied with your appearance, and you're probably not suffering a lot, but your body isn't a great source of pride or pleasure either.

If your body image is mostly positive, good for you! Given that you're reading this book, however, I suspect that there are probably still some aspects of your body image that you feel could be improved.

Next, check off all the body parts that you gave a rating of –2 or –3. These are the ones you want to be sure to work on as part of this program. If you don't have any items rated this low, then just check the ones that were rated –1. As a next step, I'd like you to move on to the assessment of thoughts that relate to your body image concerns.

Assessing Your Thoughts

You're constantly thinking, but you may not always be fully aware of your actual thoughts. However, the more you know about your thoughts, the better you can target them in treatment. The test on pages 59–62 lists some thoughts related to your looks. Of course, everyone has thoughts about their appearance at times.

Assessing Satisfaction with Body Parts

−3, dislike very much; −2, mostly dislike; −1, dislike somewhat; 0, neither like nor dislike; 1, somewhat satisfied; 2, mostly satisfied; 3, very satisfied

1. face/head _____

   a. skin (for example, color, scarring, pore size, facial hair (including eyebrows), moles, freckles, pimples) _____

   b. features (for example, eyes, nose, mouth, ears, cheekbones) _____

   c. teeth _____

   d. shape of head _____

   e. hair (for example, thickness, texture, color, cut) _____

2. neck, shoulders _____

3. arms, hands _____

4. chest, breasts _____

5. waist, stomach _____

6. buttocks, hips, thighs, legs, feet _____

7. genitals _____

8. weight, height, muscle tone _____

9. overall body hair _____

10. overall body skin _____

11. _____

12. _____

13. _____

We all notice when we have a pimple, know that we have a scar or crooked teeth, and are aware how frizzy or unruly our hair looks on a bad-hair day. In reality, most people just don't look as they would like to. But while some people can just accept their flaws and go on with their day, people with body image concerns often keep thinking about their defects and assume that these flaws have a major impact on their lives. Indeed, it's very common for someone with body image problems to feel that others are judging him or her negatively. Often the appearance flaw also leads to concerns about one's worth as a person. Therefore, the thoughts that you may have about appearance imperfections can be quite painful. As a next step, I'd like you to assess your appearance-related thoughts. Before reading on, please complete the questionnaire on pages 59–62.

Now that you've finished the questionnaire, I hope it helped you recognize which thoughts you have. It might also have given you an idea of how bothersome the thoughts are. As you probably noticed, I left some space for additional thoughts that might be related to your body image problems. Don't to get too caught up in calculating a total score, because these ratings are not based on any research, but rather on an educated guess. The main reason for looking at the ratings is to help you with goal setting.

You might have some ratings that are really high, and these are the ones we definitely want to target in this program. To ensure that we address your most distressing thoughts, you may want to put a little check mark next to all the thoughts that you gave a rating of 5 or higher. If you don't have any thoughts rated higher than 5, then just check your six or seven thoughts with the highest score. These are the ones you need to focus on. If all of your scores have the same rating, you could work on all of them. If this seems too overwhelming, just pick about six or seven thoughts to target for now.

Assessing Your Avoidance Behavior

Negative thoughts are only one way that a distorted body image manifests itself. Avoidance behavior is another. In the following section, you'll assess how many activities you are avoiding or enduring only with intense discomfort because of your body image problems. Before reading on, please complete the questionnaire on pages 63–64.

Again, you'll notice I've left space for you to fill in a couple of situations you avoid (or only tolerate with difficulty) that aren't listed. As part of this program you'll learn to reenter the situations you currently avoid and to react to them less negatively. Therefore, as a next step, put a little check mark next to all the items that you gave a rating of 5 or higher. These are the situations you want to be sure to work on as part of this program. If you don't have any items rated higher than 5, then just check the six or seven items with the highest score. If all of your items have the same rating, you could work on all of them. If this seems too overwhelming, just pick about six or seven for now to target.

Assessing Appearance-Related Thoughts

Please *circle* the number that best describes how *frequent and distressing* these thoughts and beliefs were during the past week. Don't worry too much about the exact wording of the thoughts. If you had thoughts that were similar in content, just rate those (for example, instead of "If my appearance is defective, I'm worthless," you might be thinking, "Because my nose is flawed, I'm inadequate," but the two mean essentially the same thing).

1. I believe others are thinking of my appearance.

       0   1   2   3   4   5   6   7   8   9   10
       no   moderately   very
     problem   frequent/distressing   frequent/distressing

2. The first thing people notice about me is what's wrong with my appearance.

       0   1   2   3   4   5   6   7   8   9   10
       no   moderately   very
     problem   frequent/distressing   frequent/distressing

3. I think that others are staring at or talking about me.

       0   1   2   3   4   5   6   7   8   9   10
       no   moderately   very
     problem   frequent/distressing   frequent/distressing

4. I believe others treat me differently because of my physical defects.

       0   1   2   3   4   5   6   7   8   9   10
       no   moderately   very
     problem   frequent/distressing   frequent/distressing

5. If my appearance is defective, I'm worthless.

       0   1   2   3   4   5   6   7   8   9   10
       no   moderately   very
     problem   frequent/distressing   frequent/distressing

6. If my appearance is defective, I'll end up alone and isolated.

       0   1   2   3   4   5   6   7   8   9   10
       no   moderately   very
     problem   frequent/distressing   frequent/distressing

7. If my appearance is defective, I'm helpless.

       0   1   2   3   4   5   6   7   8   9   10
       no   moderately   very
     problem   frequent/distressing   frequent/distressing

(continued)

8. No one can like me as long as I look the way I do.

   0   1   2   3   4   5   6   7   8   9   10
   no   moderately   very
   problem   frequent/distressing   frequent/distressing

9. If my appearance is defective, I'm unlovable.

   0   1   2   3   4   5   6   7   8   9   10
   no   moderately   very
   problem   frequent/distressing   frequent/distressing

10. I must look perfect.

   0   1   2   3   4   5   6   7   8   9   10
   no   moderately   very
   problem   frequent/distressing   frequent/distressing

11. My appearance has ruined my life.

   0   1   2   3   4   5   6   7   8   9   10
   no   moderately   very
   problem   frequent/distressing   frequent/distressing

12. I look defective or abnormal.

   0   1   2   3   4   5   6   7   8   9   10
   no   moderately   very
   problem   frequent/distressing   frequent/distressing

13. I hate the way I look.

   0   1   2   3   4   5   6   7   8   9   10
   no   moderately   very
   problem   frequent/distressing   frequent/distressing

14. I have to change my appearance radically.

   0   1   2   3   4   5   6   7   8   9   10
   no   moderately   very
   problem   frequent/distressing   frequent/distressing

15. I'm an unattractive person.

   0   1   2   3   4   5   6   7   8   9   10
   no   moderately   very
   problem   frequent/distressing   frequent/distressing

(continued)

16. What I look like is an important part of who I am.

    0   1   2   3   4   5   6   7   8   9   10

  no   moderately   very
problem   frequent/distressing   frequent/distressing

17. Outward appearance is a sign of the inner person.

    0   1   2   3   4   5   6   7   8   9   10

  no   moderately   very
problem   frequent/distressing   frequent/distressing

18. No one else my age looks as bad as I do.

    0   1   2   3   4   5   6   7   8   9   10

  no   moderately   very
problem   frequent/distressing   frequent/distressing

19. If I could look just the way I wish, I'd be much happier.

    0   1   2   3   4   5   6   7   8   9   10

  no   moderately   very
problem   frequent/distressing   frequent/distressing

20. People would like me less if they knew what I really look like.

    0   1   2   3   4   5   6   7   8   9   10

  no   moderately   very
problem   frequent/distressing   frequent/distressing

21. My appearance is more important than my personality, intelligence, values, skills, how I relate to others, and my performance at work or in other settings.

    0   1   2   3   4   5   6   7   8   9   10

  no   moderately   very
problem   frequent/distressing   frequent/distressing

22. If I learn to accept myself, I'll lose my motivation to look better.

    0   1   2   3   4   5   6   7   8   9   10

  no   moderately   very
problem   frequent/distressing   frequent/distressing)

23. If I looked better, my whole life would be better.

    0   1   2   3   4   5   6   7   8   9   10

  no   moderately   very
problem   frequent/distressing   frequent/distressing

(*continued*)

24. If I don't look perfect, people won't like me.

0	1	2	3	4	5	6	7	8	9	10

no
problem   moderately
frequent/distressing   very
frequent/distressing

25. If others knew what I really look like (for example, without makeup), they'd reject me.

0	1	2	3	4	5	6	7	8	9	10

no
problem   moderately
frequent/distressing   very
frequent/distressing

26. I need to look perfect in order to be accepted.

0	1	2	3	4	5	6	7	8	9	10

no
problem   moderately
frequent/distressing   very
frequent/distressing

27. If my appearance is flawed, I'm inadequate.

0	1	2	3	4	5	6	7	8	9	10

no
problem   moderately
frequent/distressing   very
frequent/distressing

28. I am ugly, because I feel ugly.

0	1	2	3	4	5	6	7	8	9	10

no
problem   moderately
frequent/distressing   very
frequent/distressing

29. People are nice to me because they feel sorry for me due to my looks.

0	1	2	3	4	5	6	7	8	9	10

no
problem   moderately
frequent/distressing   very
frequent/distressing

30.

0	1	2	3	4	5	6	7	8	9	10

no
problem   moderately
frequent/distressing   very
frequent/distressing

31.

0	1	2	3	4	5	6	7	8	9	10

no
problem   moderately
frequent/distressing   very
frequent/distressing

Situations You Are Likely to Avoid or Endure with Discomfort

Please *circle* the number that best describes *how much distress* the following situations have caused you in the past week. Perhaps you were able to tolerate the situations, but they caused you severe anxiety or shame. Or they might have been so distressing that you avoided them completely. When rating these situations, also think about *how frequently* your difficulties occurred and how they get in the way of having a good life.

1. Mirrors or reflective surfaces

    0   1   2   3   4   5   6   7   8   9   10
    no   moderately   very
    problem   severe   severe

2. Social situations where family, friends, acquaintances, and coworkers are present (for example, work, parties, family gatherings, meetings, talking in small groups, having a conversation, dating, speaking to a boss or supervisor)

    0   1   2   3   4   5   6   7   8   9   10
    no   moderately   very
    problem   severe   severe

3. Public areas (for example, stores, busy streets, restaurants, movies, buses, trains, parks, waiting in lines, public restrooms)

    0   1   2   3   4   5   6   7   8   9   10
    no   moderately   very
    problem   severe   severe

4. Intimate or close physical contact with others (for example, sexual activity, hugging, kissing, dancing, and talking closely)

    0   1   2   3   4   5   6   7   8   9   10
    no   moderately   very
    problem   severe   severe

5. Physical activities such as exercise or recreation, because of concern about appearance

    0   1   2   3   4   5   6   7   8   9   10
    no   moderately   very
    problem   severe   severe

(continued)

6. Being seen nude or with few clothes

0	1	2	3	4	5	6	7	8	9	10
no problem					moderately severe					very severe

7. Changing appearance (for example, getting a haircut)

0	1	2	3	4	5	6	7	8	9	10
no problem					moderately severe					very severe

8. Getting your picture taken, being videotaped, and so forth.

0	1	2	3	4	5	6	7	8	9	10
no problem					moderately severe					very severe

9. Discounting or avoiding compliments

0	1	2	3	4	5	6	7	8	9	10
no problem					moderately severe					very severe

10. Hiding appearance (with clothing, hairstyle, jewelry, hats, hands, body position, or makeup, and avoiding being seen without makeup, hat, etc.)

0	1	2	3	4	5	6	7	8	9	10
no problem					moderately severe					very severe

11. _____

0	1	2	3	4	5	6	7	8	9	10
no problem					moderately severe					very severe

12. _____

0	1	2	3	4	5	6	7	8	9	10
no problem					moderately severe					very severe

People engage in all kinds of behaviors to deal with their appearance concerns. In the test on pages 67–70, I'll ask you to assess the severity of your beauty rituals.

What Are Your Rituals?

- **"What's normal and what's not?"** Often, when my patients first describe their rituals in treatment or try to set goals, they say: "I've really lost touch with what's normal. I don't know how much time it should take me to put on my makeup or clothes in the morning. How long do others take in front of the mirror before they leave the house? Doesn't everyone pick at his or her pimples? Do others ask for reassurance about their appearance, too?" Especially if you have had body image concerns for a long time, it can be difficult to decide how much time you should spend on beauty-related activities. It's important, though, that you have some idea what normal behavior is, if you want to determine the severity of your problem. Therefore, I address some of the most frequently asked questions about appearance rituals here.
- **"How long should it take me to get ready?"** When getting ready in the morning, most people spend only a few seconds or minutes checking their appearance in the mirror. They rarely inspect certain body parts for extended periods of time. They usually don't change their clothes after they've picked an outfit for the day. If you have body image problems, you might spend more than an hour per day checking your appearance in the mirror, grooming, and so forth. You might change your outfits several times before deciding on one; as a result, you might even be late for work, school, or social engagements.
- **"Do others pick at their skin, too?"** While skin picking is a very common behavior, few people spend more than 10 minutes per day or experience any distress, scarring, or bleeding as a result of it. Thus, if you're spending excessive amounts of time picking your skin, or if you're very distressed as a result of your picking, I strongly recommend that you make changing this behavior part of your program.
- **"How much reassurance seeking is OK?"** Almost everyone occasionally asks a family member or friend for an opinion regarding an outfit, a new lipstick, and so forth. That's pretty common behavior. But if several times per day you ask others variations of the same appearance-related questions ("Do you notice anything unusual about my skin?" or "Can you see this pimple?"), you likely have a problem that needs to be addressed. The same is true if you keep asking questions about your appearance, although you know that the other person is already tired of responding to you.
- **"How much spending is too much?"** Whereas most of us don't mind spending a small percentage (less than 25%) of our income on clothes or beauty products, others shop till they (almost) drop. They have financial problems

because of unnecessary purchases of beauty or hair replacement products. If you run your credit card up to the limit to pay for your beauty addiction, you should certainly give problems with spending a high rating in the test on pages 67–70.

• **"Is plastic surgery OK? Someone else I know had a face lift, too. . . ."** Just about everyone would love to look movie star perfect. And since plastic surgery has become somewhat more affordable, many people choose to buy their too-good-to-be-true looks at plastic surgeons' offices. For some people with reasonably healthy body images, a visit to a plastic surgeon or dermatologist might actually enhance self-esteem. However, if you have BDD and keep looking at the mirror every few minutes planning surgeries to fix flaws that no one else can see, surgery is likely to have a negative impact on your body image. If thinking about surgeries, and perhaps even undergoing them, consumes a lot of your time (or money), you should indicate this in the test. Indeed, several of my patients couldn't pay their surgery bills, and their credit ratings suffered. Eventually, collection agencies came to get what was owed. Often they had social and relationship problems as a direct result of their spending on surgery. You also need to ask yourself honestly if you're rationally considering the potential health risks (for example, scarring) and recovery time associated with surgery. If you think you have a problem with surgery, you should indicate this with a high rating in the test.

• **"How much exercise is excessive?"** Everyone knows that moderate amounts of exercise (for example, about 30 minutes a day several times a week) are good for you. However, warning signs of problems include spending most of your free time at the gym and experiencing pain, discomfort, or prolonged fatigue after exercising. If exercise is all about impressing a mirror rather than feeling healthy or less stressed, your test score will indicate this. Before reading on, make sure you have completed the test on pages 67–70.

If this information is not enough to help you understand what is normal versus problematic behavior, ask three people you trust about their opinion or habits. Use their average time or frequency of the specific behavior that you are curious about as the norm. Then evaluate how much you deviate from this average. Obviously, the more your deviate from the average behavior, the more likely it is that you have a problem, which you should indicate in the test. Also, pay attention to the unsolicited feedback you get from people who love and care about you. If your spouse and children keep telling you that you spend too much time or money on makeup or hair replacement products, you probably do.

As you can see, I left some space so that you can include additional rituals if you like. Sometimes it's difficult to decide whether something is an unhealthy beauty compulsion that you should include on this form or just a normal habit. The amount of time you spend doing it might give you a clue. If you engage in an appearance-related behavior much more often than you would actually like to, or if the behavior starts interfering with your day-to-day activities, you

Assessing the Severity of Your Beauty Rituals

Please *circle* the number that best describes how *frequent* and *distressing* each listed appearance ritual was during the last week.

1. Comparing my appearance to others' appearance (in person, in pictures, or in the media)

   0   1   2   3   4   5   6   7   8   9   10

   no   moderately   very
   problem   frequent/distressing   frequent/distressing

2. Scrutinizing others

   0   1   2   3   4   5   6   7   8   9   10

   no   moderately   very
   problem   frequent/distressing   frequent/distressing

3. Checking or inspecting certain parts of my body

   0   1   2   3   4   5   6   7   8   9   10

   no   moderately   very
   problem   frequent/distressing   frequent/distressing

4. Measuring body part(s) or counting hairs

   0   1   2   3   4   5   6   7   8   9   10

   no   moderately   very
   problem   frequent/distressing   frequent/distressing

5. Touching or feeling body parts

   0   1   2   3   4   5   6   7   8   9   10

   no   moderately   very
   problem   frequent/distressing   frequent/distressing

6. Asking questions about my appearance over and over again, even though I understood the answer the first time

   0   1   2   3   4   5   6   7   8   9   10

   no   moderately   very
   problem   frequent/distressing   frequent/distressing

(continued)

7. Mentally reviewing past events, conversations, and actions to find out how people reacted to my appearance

   0   1   2   3   4   5   6   7   8   9   10

   no
   problem   moderately
   frequent/distressing   very
   frequent/distressing

8. Checking mirrors or other reflecting surfaces repeatedly

   0   1   2   3   4   5   6   7   8   9   10

   no
   problem   moderately
   frequent/distressing   very
   frequent/distressing

9. Washing and grooming myself longer than necessary

   0   1   2   3   4   5   6   7   8   9   10

   no
   problem   moderately
   frequent/distressing   very
   frequent/distressing

10. Spending a lot of money to improve my appearance

    0   1   2   3   4   5   6   7   8   9   10

    no
    problem   moderately
    frequent/distressing   very
    frequent/distressing

11. Tanning

    0   1   2   3   4   5   6   7   8   9   10

    no
    problem   moderately
    frequent/distressing   very
    frequent/distressing

12. Combing/cutting my hair

    0   1   2   3   4   5   6   7   8   9   10

    no
    problem   moderately
    frequent/distressing   very
    frequent/distressing

13. Applying makeup

    0   1   2   3   4   5   6   7   8   9   10

    no
    problem   moderately
    frequent/distressing   very
    frequent/distressing

(continued)

14. Shaving

    0   1   2   3   4   5   6   7   8   9   10
    no   moderately   very
    problem   frequent/distressing   frequent/distressing

15. Dieting

    0   1   2   3   4   5   6   7   8   9   10
    no   moderately   very
    problem   frequent/distressing   frequent/distressing

16. Changing my clothes

    0   1   2   3   4   5   6   7   8   9   10
    no   moderately   very
    problem   frequent/distressing   frequent/distressing

17. Using steroids

    0   1   2   3   4   5   6   7   8   9   10
    no   moderately   very
    problem   frequent/distressing   frequent/distressing

18. Exercising excessively, lifting weights

    0   1   2   3   4   5   6   7   8   9   10
    no   moderately   very
    problem   frequent/distressing   frequent/distressing

19. Skin picking

    0   1   2   3   4   5   6   7   8   9   10
    no   moderately   very
    problem   frequent/distressing   frequent/distressing

20. Pulling or plucking my hair

    0   1   2   3   4   5   6   7   8   9   10
    no   moderately   very
    problem   frequent/distressing   frequent/distressing

(continued)

21. Visiting plastic surgeons, dermatologists, or dentists to improve my appearance

    0   1   2   3   4   5   6   7   8   9   10
    no   moderately   very
    problem   frequent/distressing   frequent/distressing

22. Obtaining cosmetic surgery

    0   1   2   3   4   5   6   7   8   9   10
    no   moderately   very
    problem   frequent/distressing   frequent/distressing

23. Using medications or topical treatments to correct defects (for example, skin blemishes, baldness)

    0   1   2   3   4   5   6   7   8   9   10
    no   moderately   very
    problem   frequent/distressing   frequent/distressing

24. Reading about different methods to improve my appearance (for example, on the internet, in magazines)

    0   1   2   3   4   5   6   7   8   9   10
    no   moderately   very
    problem   frequent/distressing   frequent/distressing

25. _____

    0   1   2   3   4   5   6   7   8   9   10
    no   moderately   very
    problem   frequent/distressing   frequent/distressing

26. _____

    0   1   2   3   4   5   6   7   8   9   10
    no   moderately   very
    problem   frequent/distressing   frequent/distressing

should definitely include it on your form. Also think about how hard it would be to give up the beauty ritual. If it would be very difficult for you to stop or reduce the behavior, you may want to consider putting it on your form as well. I hope the test helps you recognize which rituals you might have. Please indicate with a check mark all the items that you gave a rating of 5 or higher. These are the rituals you definitely want to decrease as part of this program. If you don't have any items rated higher than 5, then just check your six or seven rituals with the highest score. If all of your items have the same rating, you can work on all of them. If there are too many and this seems too overwhelming, just pick about six or seven for now to target.

After you've identified the body parts that trouble you and your thoughts, avoidance behaviors, and rituals, it's helpful to write down even more details about them in notes next to the items. If you run out of space, use an extra piece of paper. For example, if one of your rituals is applying makeup or cleaning your face, think about whether you have to get it done in a particular order or in a special way. If you've noticed that you avoid certain poses, ask yourself: Does this occur in all situations or only when I'm around people who intimidate me? If you check your appearance in any way (through measuring, mirror checking, touching, etc.), think about how long it usually takes you. How often do you have to repeat it? If you're not sure, just observe yourself for a couple of days, then write the information down. Try to learn as much as you can about your problems. The more you know about them, the easier it will be to change them.

Your Long-Term Goals

Once you have a pretty good understanding of what's bothering you, it's time to start setting goals. Your goals will ultimately help you plan your self-help program. When people first come into treatment, I always ask them what they hope to accomplish as part of their therapy. Often the response is "I want to feel better about my appearance." Although this is certainly a good start, I always press them for additional, more specific goals, especially as they relate to thoughts and behaviors; for example, "I want to learn to evaluate my thoughts and discover alternative ways of thinking" or "I want to reduce my mirror checking from 90 to 5 minutes per day" or "I want to be able to go to work without makeup." You get the idea: Most of the goals that you set for yourself should be pretty specific. The best goals are *measurable*, so that you can easily tell whether you reached them (for example, "reduce checking time by 85 minutes" or "no more plastic surgery"). Also, the better defined your goal, the easier it will be to work toward it. Another important feature of a good goal is that it should be within your control. For example, a goal such as "I want to have blemish-free, perfectly white, smooth skin" is not helpful, because you have only limited control over what your skin looks like (to a large degree it's determined by your genes).

By completing the assessment forms, you've already taken the first step in the right direction: You've identified the problems. Next you'll have to reword these problems into goals. So, for example, if your problem was a preoccupation with your nose and the resulting avoidance of public areas (for example, restaurants, trains, parks, waiting in lines), one of your long-term goals might be to be able to go to these places again on a daily basis.

Before you write down your own long-term goals, take a look at Ada's worksheets. Ada, a 42-year-old marketing manager, is married and has two children. When I first met her, she was very preoccupied with her skin (particularly her facial skin). She also had some less severe concerns about hair on her legs. First, she completed all the assessments and transferred the problems that related to the skin to a Long-Term Goals Worksheet (page 73). Next, she reworded her problems as goals. She then completed an additional worksheet (page 74) for the problems she had with the hair on her legs.

After you've reviewed Ada's worksheets, try to complete your own (page 75). Start by reviewing all items that you've marked with a check in the assessment section. Write them all in the appropriate categories. If you're preoccupied with more than one body part or body area, use several worksheets and fill out one for each problem area. Also, don't hesitate to use several worksheets if you run out of space listing the thoughts or behaviors related to your particular problem.

Which Problem Area Should You Work on First?

If you have completed several worksheets for different problem areas, you should now arrange your worksheets in order of importance. I suggest you start with the worksheet that lists the problem that bothers you the most, maybe because it interferes with doing things you'd like to do or because it causes you problems at school or work. Working on problems that interfere with your life keeps you motivated, because you know that the reward is high once you succeed.

Nevertheless, there are some exceptions to this rule: If you have any worksheets that include plans for irreversible procedures such as plastic surgery, major dental or dermatological interventions, or self-surgery, you should focus on these issues first. This is very important, because even if the body parts for which you're planning these procedures are not causing you a huge problem yet, they might really start troubling you after you've had the procedure. Similarly, if you have a problem with skin picking that could result in severe tissue damage, it's a good idea to focus on this right away.

Sometimes my patients tell me the preoccupation with one body part and related avoidance behaviors and rituals are so severe that they're afraid to work on this problem area so early in the program. In this case, I recommend working on a somewhat less distressing problem first. You can still approach the really dif-

Long-Term Goals Worksheet: Ada (I)

(Include only symptoms with a check mark)

My problem area:

Preoccupation with skin (esp. facial blemishes and large pores on face)

Related thoughts:

3. *I think that others are staring at or talking about me.*

5. *If my appearance is defective, I'm worthless.*

9. *If my appearance is defective, I'm unlovable.*

Related avoidance behavior:

2. *Social situations where family, friends, acquaintances, coworkers are present (esp. meetings at work, church)*

10. *Hiding appearance (esp. with makeup, concealer)*

Related rituals:

1. *Comparing my appearance to others' appearance*

5. *Touching or feeling body parts*

6. *Asking questions about my appearance over and over again, even though I understood the answer the first time (esp. husband)*

9. *Washing and grooming myself longer than necessary*

13. *Applying make up over and over again*

My long-term goals for this problem:

1. *I will learn ways to evaluate and perhaps change the thoughts listed above.*

2. *I will not avoid any situations where family, friends, acquaintances, coworkers are present.*

3. *I will not hide my face with makeup.*

4. *I will not compare my appearance (esp. skin) to others.*

5. *I will not ask my husband "Do you see a pimple?" at all.*

6. *I will wash my face only twice a day for 30 seconds.*

Long-Term Goals Worksheet: Ada (II)

(Include only symptoms with a check mark)

My problem area:

Legs: mainly hair

Related thoughts:

3.   I think that others are staring at or talking about me.

20.   People would like me less if they knew what I really looked like (because I always cover my legs, they don't know what I look like).

Related avoidance behavior:

10.   Hiding appearance with clothing

Related rituals:

14.   Excessive shaving

My long-term goals for this problem:

1.   I will learn ways to evaluate and perhaps change the thoughts listed above.

2.   I will not hide my legs with clothing.

3.   I will shave my legs only every other day.

Long-Term Goals Worksheet

(Include only symptoms with a check mark)

My problem area:

Related thoughts:

Related avoidance behavior:

Related rituals:

My long-term goals for this problem:

ficult ones later, once you gained a little bit of confidence. Having said all this, most of my patients end up starting with a problem area that's highly important to them. Sometimes several goals seem equally important. If that's the case for you, don't worry, just pick one; you'll get to the other ones later.

Order of Goals for Major Problem Areas

1.
2.
3.
4.

You'll start your program by working on the negative thoughts related to your most troubling problem area. You'll work on those thoughts alone for a couple of weeks before you add exposure exercises related to your most troubling problem area. Next you'll cut down your rituals. Having attained some of the cognitive skills described in Chapter 5 before you attempt to change your behavior will make your exposure and response prevention exercises much easier.

Ada organized her goals as follows: She first tackled some of the negative thoughts related to the preoccupation with her skin. After 2 weeks, she did not believe as strongly that others were staring at her skin. Because her beliefs had changed, it was much easier to address her avoidance behavior, and she started exposing herself to social situations. After having mastered a couple of exposures, she also learned to decrease her ritualistic behaviors, such as the excessive makeup application. Your program will look very similar. You'll start working on cognitive strategies before you move on to exposure and response prevention.

Although some of your goals in therapy can perhaps be addressed with only exposure or just ritual prevention, many of your exercises will need to include both. In other words, often your goal will be as follows: I will do exposure to X situation, which I usually avoid, and without engaging in ritual Y. Whereas the cognitive techniques and exposure practices might reduce the fear of the situation, the best way to reduce your compulsive behaviors is with response prevention. Thus, you'll ultimately get the most out of this program if you are flexible and learn to combine your work on thoughts, exposure to avoided situations, and ritual prevention. Ada found that her cognitive skills and the related changes in beliefs helped her cut down the amount of time she spent applying makeup before leaving the house and while she was out. At times when she left the house, she felt anxious and wanted to avoid and ritualize. However, instead of giving in to those urges, she used her new cognitive skills to talk herself through the situations. Eventually, she even learned to go out without doing any rituals at all. You can be just as successful as Ada, and the worksheets in the following chapters will guide you through this process.

What If You Find Yourself Dragging Your Feet?

If you're having a tough time getting started, review your cost–benefit analysis from Chapter 3. Getting out of a rut and starting something new is always difficult. But keep in mind that you are going to set your goals in such a manner that your anxiety remains manageable. This way it's highly likely that you'll reach those goals. The progress you see along the way will fill you with a sense of pride and accomplishment. Many of the activities you're dreading right now will become more enjoyable or even fun, so the work you do will be self-reinforcing. The investment you make is relatively small in comparison to what you have to gain. Get going . . . it's worth it!

Practice, Practice, Practice

The ratings on the assessment tests in this chapter can give you an idea of how long the program might take. On average, the program will take about 12 weeks. However, if you have only low scores and few negative thoughts, limited avoidance behaviors, and few rituals, you might be able to finish the program in 10 weeks. On the other hand, if you have many high ratings, you might need a bit more time, let's say 16 weeks or more. Higher ratings translate into a longer program because you'll start gradually and conquer one problem at a time.

Sometimes it is helpful to spend extra time on a section if you feel that there's more you could learn. You don't need to rush through the program. The program works best if you practice every day. Many of my former patients have set aside 45 minutes to an hour a day to improve their body image. This sounds like a lot of time, but you'll reach your goals sooner and have less chance of relapse. It's very simple: The more you practice, the more you'll improve.

What If You Don't Feel Like Working on the Program?

Even though you know you should practice every day, there may be days when you don't feel like it. This may be because you're too anxious or you just aren't motivated. It's important not to get discouraged in these situations. Just try to figure out why you didn't complete your practice. If you're too anxious to try a particular short-term goal, you might have to set a slightly easier one. It's better to attempt an easier task and go a little slower than to make no progress at all. If you just don't feel up to working on your program, reread Chapter 3 and ask yourself about the pros and cons of continuing with this work. Even if you are motivated and making progress, it's a good idea occasionally to review what you've learned. For example, you could spend about 20 minutes a week revisiting material you've already covered.

Evaluate Your Progress

Monitoring of your progress is an important part of the program. A good way to monitor your improvement is to retake the tests you took at the beginning of this chapter, once every month. You should start seeing changes, at the latest, after you have worked on this program for 8 weeks. Most people see improvement sooner. In Chapters 6 and 7, you will also learn how to use your discomfort ratings to monitor your progress with respect to reaching your short-term goals. You are done with a particular short-term or long-term goal after you score a low rating on the discomfort scale. Similarly, your program is probably nearing its end when your scores on individual items in the tests in this chapter are in the 0–3 range.

Realism: A Key to Success

Optimism and conviction are important to staying actively involved with this program, but they shouldn't preclude realism. Keeping these two caveats in mind will ensure that your expectations are reasonable and prevent you from being discouraged by failure to meet lofty goals.

Urges to Avoid and to Ritualize Will Persist

The urge to ritualize or to avoid will persist for quite some time, even if you understand that these behaviors are irrational. They are a little bit like old habits that are sometimes hard to break. Remember that change takes time, and the urges to ritualize and to avoid will weaken if you keep teaching yourself that you can handle trigger situations *without* the rituals.

Be Realistic: Expect Ups and Downs

There is no magic cure or quick fix for body image problems, and, especially in the beginning, you will not always be successful with your new strategies. There will be days when you are doing great. But there will also be days when you feel stuck and things get temporarily worse. Realize that these setbacks are a normal part of the process. Hang in there, and don't let these obstacles stop you. Try to use setbacks as learning experiences that can teach you how to prevent problems in the future. There is no such thing as smooth progress; therefore, it is important to look at the long-term picture rather than making day-to-day comparisons.

It is very likely that this program will help you. However, if you do get stuck over the course of the program, I'll provide you with hints that will help you move along. For example, occasionally I come across patients who are repeating their exposure exercises as they should but don't really get more comfortable over time. This is rare, but it is usually due to their engagement in some sort of ritualistic or safety behavior while doing the exposure. This prevents them from learning that things would have turned out just fine without any rituals; therefore, the anxiety never lessens. Over the course of the program, I'll teach you how to avoid these glitches, and to address them when they occur.

I've occasionally had patients who were discouraged with their progress, although objectively they were actually doing quite well. You may not recognize your progress, or you might discount it, especially if you're depressed. Some discounting may be linked to perfectionistic standards and dichotomous thinking: "If I'm not completely better, progress is irrelevant." If you have these kind of thoughts, strategies outlined in Chapter 5 that address all-or-nothing thinking might be helpful.

Chapter 5

Managing Your Thoughts

As explained in Chapter 3, the messages that run through your mind determine how you feel and what you do. Every time you feel anxious, discouraged, or self-conscious about your looks, it's the result of negative thinking. But our thoughts aren't always trustworthy. The fact that negative thoughts about your appearance often come into your mind doesn't mean that they are true. Indeed, they may be absolutely illogical, inaccurate, even bizarre—and they're certainly not helpful.

In this chapter, I'll help you see this for yourself. You start by learning to recognize illogical and self-defeating thinking, then learning to change these negative thoughts and painful feelings. If you're now thinking that your thoughts aren't the problem ("Other people might just have a little problem with their thinking, and they can benefit from this psychological stuff, but I really have a *physical* problem! There's something wrong with the way I look!"), you might be surprised to know that I hear the same protest from almost every new patient. In fact, after the first session of the first BDD group that I ran, several patients called me to say they couldn't come back to future sessions. Why? "Because everybody else in the group looked fine; they just have a psychological problem. I'm the only one who *looks* weird!" You, too, have probably been convinced that all you need is a change in the way you look. But keep in mind that this belief is the core of your problem, and this is why your thinking needs fine-tuning: You have started to believe things that aren't based on reality.

Your Negative Feelings Are Caused by Your Thoughts

As introduced in Chapter 3, one of the basic assumptions of CBT is that how you interpret a situation affects how you feel. In other words, you aren't reacting with anxiety or sadness to certain events or situations; rather, you are reacting to your *interpretations* of these situations. Let me give you an example. Let's say you are at a party chatting with some friends. All of a sudden, you realize that someone keeps looking at you. What kinds of thoughts run through your mind? Just try to pick one of these interpretations:

   a. He's interested in our conversation.
   b. He thinks I look strange.
   c. He's looking in my direction but not really looking at me (that is, he's daydreaming).
   d. He's interested in me.

If you picked *a* or *d*, you probably feel pretty good as a result of your interpretation. You might look back at the observer and smile. Or you might get more animated and confident in the conversation with your friends. If you picked *c*, you likely feel neutral and just keep doing whatever you are doing. If you picked *b*, however, you'll probably feel anxious, and you may even change your behavior (for example, turn your back to the observer) as a result of this thought. All of these interpretations are equally likely, and the one you picked created your reality and changed how you felt and behaved. The same relationship applies to most situations in life. It's not really what's happening to you that causes you to feel sad, self-confident, anxious, or neutral. It's how you interpret what's happening.

Likewise, when you look in the mirror, you're not just getting input from your retina and visual cortex; you're also *interpreting your reflection* in some way. If you look at your nose and decide that it looks *disfigured* because it's a little bumpy, you feel sad and discouraged. If you decide that although your nose isn't perfect, it's OK, and that you really love your eyes, you'll feel good or relatively neutral as a result of your mirror inspection.

It's not your appearance that's causing a problem, but your evaluation of it. Your appearance evaluation fluctuates based on your mood or thoughts of the moment. Let's assume you had a good day in school or at work, you're in a happy mood, and you're checking out your body. You determine that on a scale of 100 you may be a 50—and that's OK. Next, let's pretend you watch *Baywatch* and compare yourself to the superbeautiful cast. Now you're feeling pretty insecure, and you might decide that looking like a "50" is disastrous. Your appearance didn't change, but the way you thought about it changed. Again, it's the meaning you attach to your appearance, and not your appearance itself, that causes your negative feelings.

Your Thoughts May Be Unhelpful or False

Often your interpretations of situations are correct, but sometimes they're exaggerated or even absolutely false. Preoccupied with her large "elephant" ears, Nastasia was quick to assume that others would reject her because of this flaw. One day after class, she tried to strike up a conversation with one of her classmates. When he excused himself after a few minutes, Nastasia assumed that he'd cut the conversation short because he didn't like the way she looked. In reality, he could have left for several reasons:

- He was pressed for time.
- He wasn't interested in the conversation topic.
- He was characteristically shy or socially anxious.
- He felt sick, tired, or hungry that day.
- He considered conversation a waste of time.
- He was worried about something.

These are just a few of the many possibilities that Nastasia didn't consider. If you honestly reviewed a situation in which you drew a similar conclusion, you would probably find that you, too, assume that others are reacting negatively to your appearance, without even considering other, possibly more likely explanations for their behavior. The questions is why so many of us come up with these hurtful explanations for benign events.

Why Do You Assume the Worst?

You always have a stream of thoughts running through your mind. They're reactions and interpretations to whatever is happening to and around you. Sometimes the thoughts are neutral or pleasant; at other times, they are self-defeating or unpleasant. They can make you sad, anxious, or ashamed. If you have a body image problem, chances are that most thoughts related to your appearance are negative. They just pop up and cause you to feel bad. The fact that they emerge without any effort on your part is why Dr. Aaron Beck, a highly respected cognitive therapist, named them *automatic thoughts*.

Automatic thoughts are situation-specific, so they can change somewhat depending on where you are and whose company you keep. But they always end up making you feel bad. Why is this the case for you? Everyone has appearance flaws and occasionally thinks about them. How come some people can just let those thoughts pass through their mind, without experiencing the shame and humiliation with which you might be struggling?

It all comes down to the much deeper beliefs that underlie your automatic thoughts. Your thoughts are influenced by the beliefs you hold about yourself, your future, and the world around you. However, unlike automatic thoughts, which may adjust from one situation to the next, these deeper level beliefs are very broad and rigid. In her book *Cognitive Therapy: Basics and Beyond,* Dr. Judith Beck describes how beliefs or assumptions may be expressed like rules, in the form of "if . . . then" statements. Several of my patients believe "If I'm not perfectly beautiful, I'm absolutely hideous." Holding on to a belief like that influences your thoughts, feelings, and behavior every day. It's hard to tolerate even the smallest appearance flaw. Beliefs like this can be buried so deep that you're not fully aware of them. Later in this book, I show you how to uncover and change them. For now, let's take a look at a few examples of the beliefs I've come across over the years.

Typical Beliefs of People with Body Image Concerns

- If my appearance is defective, I'm worthless as a person.
- If my appearance is defective, I'll always be alone.
- If I looked better, my whole life would be better.
- If I don't look perfect, people won't like me.
- If others knew what I really look like (for example, without makeup), they'd reject me.
- I need to look perfect to be accepted.
- If my appearance is flawed, I am inadequate.
- I'm ugly because I feel ugly.

Several of these assumptions contain the idea that appearance is central to being happy or loved and accepted. In other beliefs, appearance and self-worth have become interwoven. Many of the assumptions contain perfectionistic ideas, and some contain the idea that control over appearance leads to control over feelings. You probably developed these beliefs while growing up; thus, over the years, they have been influenced by your family, cultural values, the media, and possibly even traumatic life experiences.

Any of the beliefs listed will influence what you think in any situation you encounter. They'll make it hard for you to accept yourself as you are. This will make you feel sad, anxious, or embarrassed and might even impact how you behave.

And what if they're not true? If your beliefs are false or exaggerated, your expectations and automatic thoughts in specific situations will be inaccurate. But you'll still feel bad when they arise. The next step, below, is to learn how to recognize and change negative automatic thoughts in specific situations. Later (in Chapter 8) I explain how to identify and change deeper-level beliefs.

Identifying Your Negative Thoughts

If you're going to eliminate negative thoughts, naturally you have to be able to identify them first. This may be quite easy for you, or it could be very challenging. You might think, "I'm not sure what I'm thinking; I just feel awful about the way I look." Don't worry; identifying your negative thoughts, like almost everything in life, gets easier with practice.

Using Thought Records

The most important next step is for you to start focusing on your thoughts and to write them down. You can either make photocopies of the worksheet on the facing page, Thought Record, or buy yourself a small notebook and make up your own thought record, as long as you follow the format I suggest. The goal is to spend a minimum of 20–30 minutes a day during the coming week on your thought records.

It's best to complete the Thought Record right after you've had a negative thought. Because these thoughts can occur anywhere, you should take your notebook or Thought Record forms with you wherever you go. Many of my patients take them to work and on vacation. Sometimes, however, you'll be in social or other situations in which working on a Thought Record would be inappropriate. In those cases, it's OK to delay writing down the thoughts, but don't wait too long, because you might forget important details.

If you don't have any thoughts in the next few days that make you feel uncomfortable, just imagine a future situation that might be difficult for you. Chapter 4 might help you to identify the types of situations you should watch out for. Or try to remember a recent situation that made you feel bad. Remember the situation as vividly as you can, then complete the Thought Record.

In the first section, "Situations," briefly describe the situation that triggered the negative thought. Just a few words are enough. In the second section, describe the thoughts. Write them down word for word; don't pretty them up. So, don't change the thought "I'm hideous!" to "I was thinking that I'm not very attractive." Also, don't worry about spelling or grammar. In the third section, describe how the thought made you feel.

The example on page 86 is from Amy, who was thinking about going swimming on a hot summer day. But she first had to deal with some thoughts that got in her way.

You might be thinking that you really don't want to write your negative, appearance-related thoughts down every day. They're awful, and writing them

Thought Record

Situation:

Thoughts:

Feelings:

Thought Record: Amy

Situation:

Thinking about going swimming.

Thoughts:

It will be really weird if I run into my classmates and I have no makeup on.

They'll think I look sick and pale.

They'll stare at my small breasts.

If Jack is there, he'll find out what I really look like. He'll be so disappointed.

Feelings:

Anxious, frustrated

Adapted by permission of the publisher and author from Judith S. Beck, *Cognitive Therapy: Basics and Beyond* (Guilford Press, © 1995).

down will just make you feel worse. You may not want to spend any more time thinking about this than you already do. It's true that monitoring your thoughts initially might be a challenge, because I'm asking you to focus on something that is actually quite painful for you, and you don't yet have the skills to cope. But let me assure you that writing these thoughts down is a good investment in your future. If at any point you lose the motivation to continue with thought monitoring, reread the sections on the costs and benefits of this program in Chapter 3. Yes, for a short period of time it may be difficult to do this exercise, but in the long term, most of my patients have found it extremely helpful. So even if you don't feel like it, use all your willpower to keep monitoring your thoughts. It's worth it.

When You Have Trouble Identifying Your Thoughts

If you have trouble identifying your thoughts, look for a change in the way you feel. Many of my new patients find it easier to detect a change in their mood than to detect negative thoughts. So if you notice that your mood plummets, ask yourself: "What was I just thinking? What kinds of thoughts were running through my mind?" If you aren't sure, ask yourself, "What did this particular situation mean to me?" The thoughts we're looking for often begin with "He/she/they will think . . . ," "I'm . . . ," "I will . . . ," or "I'm going to . . . ," Also keep on the lookout for emotionally loaded words like *ugly, disfigured, hideous.*

Also, pay attention to physiological changes. For example, if your heart suddenly starts beating rapidly or your face gets flushed, you might just have had an anxiety-provoking thought.

Similarly, notice when you change your behavior or experience urges to modify your actions. Examine your thinking if you suddenly interrupt eye contact or experience a strong desire to escape from a social situation. It's quite possible that all of these are indicators for self-defeating thoughts.

Finally, go back to Chapter 4, where you identified your problem areas and the situations with which you are struggling. Whenever you are confronted with these, you should be particularly watchful for negative thoughts.

When You Have Trouble Defining Your Feelings

Sometimes people have problems labeling their negative emotions. These are the most common ones that I've come across in people with body image concerns, so if you aren't sure how you are feeling, you might benefit from looking at the following list of feelings brought on by negative thoughts:

- Anxious, scared, tense, worried
- Embarrassed, ashamed, humiliated, insulted

- Sad, unhappy, defeated, gloomy, hopeless, insecure, rejected, lonely, neglected, disappointed, hurt
- Envious, jealous
- Frustrated, irritable, disgusted, angry, hostile, annoyed

Identifying Thinking Errors

By now, you know that not everything you think is true. Thoughts are only thoughts, not facts. Therefore, it's important to be able to find out whether your thoughts are useful and true or unhelpful and distorted. A good technique to accomplish this goal is to check your thoughts for certain self-defeating cognitive biases. Even highly intelligent people often have these biases in their thinking, and many mental health professionals have written about them. I found the descriptions of thinking errors by Dr. Judith Beck* particularly helpful, but I've modified them a little to make them more relevant to body image concerns.

Types of Distorted Thinking

You may realize that you commit many of the errors described on the next few pages, but understand that this doesn't mean your problem is so severe that this book can't help you. For example, in the middle of a presentation she was giving at work, a woman noticed a typo on one of her handouts. Within about 3 minutes, her thinking spanned about three or four of the cognitive errors I've listed. I was this person, so be assured, it's pretty normal to have biases in your thinking. But just because all of us have these tendencies doesn't mean that they're helpful!

Also keep in mind that many of your negative thoughts might contain more than one cognitive error. For example, the thought, "If I go to the party looking like that, Morgan will think that I look like a freak!" contains the errors fortune telling, mind reading, and labeling.

All-or-Nothing Thinking: Model or Monster?

All-or-nothing thinking means you think in such extremes that you see things as falling into one of only two categories. Everything is either black or white. There are no shades of gray. This kind of thinking shows up as the tendency to judge beauty that falls short of perfect as absolutely hideous. If you engage in this type of thinking, you may categorize yourself as either beautiful or ugly. Usually the beautiful category is narrow and therefore hard to achieve. The ugly cate-

---

*Judith S. Beck, *Cognitive Therapy: Basics and Beyond* (Guilford Press, 1995); the descriptions of thinking errors are adapted by permission of the publisher and author.

gory, on the other hand, is huge and very easy to attain. There is no such thing as looking OK, because you are either gorgeous or hideous. Not surprisingly, this style of thinking can cause you to feel sad, anxious, or disappointed.

All-or-nothing thinking is often associated with having excessively high standards. Consider Zora, who thought, "Men are attracted only to pretty women, and I'm not one of them." Unfortunately for Zora, pretty meant looking like the women in the fashion magazines. I thought Zora was actually quite attractive, and certainly above average looking, but she didn't look like a supermodel. Holding such extreme beliefs about what's pretty and what's not caused her to feel hopeless about her future. Another patient of mine, Eddie, held the belief, "If my hair isn't absolutely perfect, I look ugly." This belief caused him to invest a lot of time, money, and energy in his hair. But not surprisingly, like all of us, he often had to face days when his hair "didn't look right." Whenever this was the case, he felt hideous and was self-conscious around others. Of course, other people probably wouldn't have noticed a difference in his hair, and even if they had, they certainly couldn't have cared less. Thus, all this anxiety was caused not by reality but by Eddie's mental magic. When Eddie and I started discussing his all-or-nothing thinking related to his hair, he admitted that he thought in extremes in other areas of his life as well. He told me: "Well, on the one hand, being a bit extreme has helped me. For example, I always worked very hard in school and never would have turned in an assignment that was imperfect. So I always had good grades. But, of course, having those high standards meant that I always had to work really hard, even on things that are not very important. This costs me a lot of time. What's worse, it's hard to relax and enjoy life if your standards are so high and your thinking is so extreme. For example, recently I took an art class, just for fun, and I was painting this picture. I called my picture 'Underwater World,' and it had lots of beautiful fish and plants on it. But it had this one little yellow fish . . . and I hated the shape and color of this little fish. Even though the fish was small, I threw out the whole picture because it wasn't perfect."

Do you engage in all-or-nothing thinking? If so, write down some examples in the space below. Given that you are struggling with your appearance, make sure you come up with some examples related to how you look. But if you remember examples in other areas, feel free to put them down as well, because it's good for you to examine your overall mode of thinking.

"Should" Statements

You have strict rules about the way things "should be," and you overestimate how bad it will be if something deviates from your expectations. Of course, most of us agree that certain rules are necessary and helpful in organizing our lives. For example, most of us would think that the rule "I shouldn't cheat" is in general pretty reasonable. However, if your rule is "I should always look perfect," you're creating a standard too high to achieve. As a matter of fact, not even the highly paid models you see on magazine covers could attain this. Although you might have developed this rule to motivate yourself, the effect of having these unattainable standards is that you feel pressure, shame, guilt, and self-loathing. *Musts* and *have-to*s are just as tricky. I often hear from my patients, "I have to work out every day," which, of course, is difficult for almost everyone to do. Therefore, they fall short of their own expectations and feel lazy as a result. So, it's probably a good idea to watch out for any thoughts or statements that contain words like *should, must, ought,* and *have to.*

Do you engage in should statements? If so, write down some examples in the space below.

_____

_____

_____

_____

Mind Reading

Whenever you mind-read, you make assumptions that you know what other people are thinking. And because you are so sure about what the other person thinks, you don't even bother to check it out. Specifically, you might believe others are thinking badly about your looks. You believe that others share your view of the perceived defect—that they notice it and are appalled by the way you look. It doesn't even occur to you that the other person might have thought something neutral or positive about your appearance, or might not have thought about your appearance at all. Therefore, attention from others often makes you feel self-conscious, angry, or anxious. Of course, people sometimes do make negative judgments about one another. But this probably occurs less often than you think. In many cases, your theories about what others are thinking about your appearance are either wrong or blown out of proportion.

Cooper is a good-looking businessman. He is not only successful but also has an infectious and very likable personality. Although he goes tanning quite often, he is worried about his skin being too pale. He holds the belief, "When people look at me, they think I look weird." He would like to be in a relationship, but whenever he notices a man looking at him, this belief kicks in. He then loses his confidence and avoids eye contact. Unfortunately, Cooper's skills as a mind reader are somewhat lacking, to say the least, and his friends often tell him that he misunderstands why he gets so much attention. It's not because other people consider him unattractive. Indeed, the opposite is true.

When Gordon's classmate failed to acknowledge him on a nice summer day at the beach, he immediately turned on his mind-reading skills. "She pretends she didn't see me because she's embarrassed to talk to me in front of her friends. She probably thinks I look like a geek. This wouldn't have happened if I was more muscular!" Gordon instantly felt bitter and decided to avoid the girl in the future. Just a few minutes later, he found out she really hadn't seen him, and as soon as she did, she called out his name and then introduced him to her friends when he went over to her. All his disappointment and anger was for nothing, but Gordon was ruled by the belief that his looks revealed his inadequacy!

Do you read minds? If so, write down some examples in the space below.

_____

_____

_____

_____

Fortune Telling

If you are fortune telling, you might predict a dismal future because of your looks, without considering more likely and less catastrophic outcomes. It's very common for my patients to expect to be turned down for dates or promotions because of their looks. They often make predictions that they they'll never get married because of a "wrinkled face" or a "bumpy nose." They often foresee that they won't enjoy a party or other social event. Because they are so sure that events will turn out negatively or even catastrophically, they often end up avoiding them. This way they never get a chance to experience how it would have been just fine if they had only gone to check it out. Usually people have no objective evidence on which to base their negative expectations for the future. So, if you find yourself predicting that your future will be gloomy or that things will just turn out to be terrible, watch out for the fortune teller error.

Do you engage in fortune telling? If so, write down some examples in the space below.

_____

_____

_____

_____

Personalization (Self-Absorption)

Personalization is the tendency to consider negative or even irrelevant events as having something (negative) to do with you, rather than considering all the different factors that might have contributed to a situation. For example, Cameron thought: "The waitress was so unfriendly because she didn't like my looks." It didn't even occur to him that the waitress might have been tired, sad about something that happened earlier that day, had a headache, or had aching feet. If you personalize, attention from others often makes you feel embarrassed or ashamed. Fabian's problem with personalization and self-absorption was even worse. He was so convinced that other people were always thinking of his nose that he felt ashamed and personally insulted whenever others touched their own face. He told me, "I know that they're thinking about my nose. They're trying to tell me something when they touch their nose. Even if it's subconscious, they're still trying to tell me that my nose is too long." Because he managed to link almost every gesture someone else made to his nose, he often felt mocked and rejected. It didn't even occur to him to consider that other people's noses might have itched or that they touched their nose whenever they felt nervous. By the time he came for treatment, he was almost completely isolated, because he constantly got angry with others for mistreating him.

Asha also was an expert in personalization. One day she had a blind date she met through a newspaper ad. Although they both seemed to have a pretty good time while they were out, he never called afterward. Asha thought: "He probably didn't call back because of my crooked teeth!" She didn't consider that he might have a fear of getting involved or felt intimidated because he earned less money than she did.

Do you personalize? If so, write down some examples in the space below.

_____

_____

_____

_____

Emotional Reasoning

You think something is true because it feels true, and you just take your emotions as evidence of the truth. Emotional reasoning explains why your body image can change after you hear a critical comment about your appearance or eat a bag of potato chips. Your actual appearance has not really changed, but you may think you look fat because you feel full. My patients often tell me, "Yes, I know that many people have told me I look fine, but I still feel ugly. . . ." In other words, what they are saying is "I feel ugly; therefore, I am ugly."

You've probably noticed that your mood impacts how you feel (or actually think) about your looks. Your mood is like the music in the movies; it sets the stage for your interpretation of events. If the music is dramatic, you're more likely to read something into an otherwise harmless gesture or event. So if you're having a good day, your self-talk is more likely to be lenient and forgiving as far as your appearance imperfections go. But what if you're feeling lousy? You might feel bad about something entirely unrelated to your appearance, such as a negative evaluation at school or work. Once you start feeling ashamed, anxious, or disgusted, your busy mind goes on a search for other topics associated with these emotions. And voilà! There are your body image concerns! In other words, when you're already feeling self-conscious, it's pretty easy to remember all the other things, such as your small breasts, short stature, or crooked teeth, that usually make you feel ashamed. Your body has become an emotional dumping ground, and all your negative energy—no matter where it originally came from—gets focused there.

Do you engage in emotional reasoning? If so, write down some examples in the space below.

_____

_____

_____

_____

Labeling

Labeling means you put a label on yourself that is unhelpful, usually heavily emotionally loaded, and inaccurate. You may actually dislike only a couple of your features or body parts. But by attaching this label to yourself, you're no longer talking about these specifics; rather, you're making a global statement about your appearance or personality. There is a difference between saying to yourself that you have a pimple on your right cheek and calling yourself "zit face." Judging yourself in such a global and harsh way makes you feel sad, ashamed, and hopeless. My patients, who generally look normal or even quite attractive, have come up with all sorts of self-defeating labels, including *disgusting, disfigured, ugly, pig nose, repulsive, freak, hideous, revolting,* and so forth.

Do you engage in labeling? If so, write down some examples in the space below.

_____

_____

_____

_____

Selective Attention and Magnification

Marsha is a 37-year-old police detective. She's well respected by her colleagues, seems assertive, is the mother of two children, and looks attractive with her tall build and short red hair. Indeed, she appears successful all around. However, Marsha tells me, "My colleagues would never know it, but my self-esteem is actually quite low. I always find fault with myself, no matter what others tell me. My flaw detector works round the clock. . . . One day I think my eyelids are droopy, then my chin is too small, my pores are too large, and so forth. Lately I've been very worried about wrinkles on my forehead. What's worse, I used to enjoy the beach, but I've not been able to go since my kids were born. I'd love to take the kids. But I just hate those stretch marks and the cellulite, so I won't go."

Marsha has a problem with selectively attending to everything she dislikes. Selective attention means that you notice and remember certain things more than others. It can cause you to pay too much attention to little flaws, therefore missing the big picture. As I described earlier, it is a lot easier to attend to and recall events that are in line with your beliefs. So if you believe you look unattractive, it's a lot easier to remember when you got teased than when someone paid you a compliment.

Selective attention might also play a role in what you see when you look in the mirror. If you're dissatisfied with your appearance, it's likely that you pay a lot of attention to any body part you consider imperfect. Other people who aren't as appearance-obsessed are able to disregard minor imperfections because they don't believe they are really important enough to warrant so much attention. The problem with paying too much attention to something is that it starts looking funny after a while. If I keep staring at my nose long enough, it eventually appears huge and obvious.

You may not only selectively attend to imperfections but you may also go so far as to magnify your flaws. For example, if you have a pimple, you think: "Oh my God, how horrible! How disgusting! Everybody will be staring at me!" And the pimple will appear gigantic and grotesque.

Do you engage in selective attention or magnification? If so, write down some examples in the space below.

_____

_____

_____

_____

Discounting the Positives

Marsha, described earlier, not only had a problem with selectively attending to her flaws, but also she didn't pay any attention to her beautiful features. You might just do the same and filter out anything that is good or, even worse, you might distort it, so that in the end it winds up being negative: "She was only nice because she felt sorry for me"; "It went OK because it was so dark that he didn't see my acne scars"; "Yes, she told me I look good. But she knows how much I struggle with my looks. So she probably just said it because she wanted me to feel better"; "Yes, he did pay me a compliment. But I was also wearing a lot of makeup that day. If he knew what I really look like, he never would have said that I'm pretty!" Discounting anything positive that comes your way not only prevents you from appreciating or enjoying compliments or other nice events but it can also lead you to maintain a false belief, despite the contradictory evidence right under your nose.

Do you ever discount your positive attributes? If so, write down some examples in the space below.

_____

_____

_____

_____

A Test Run: Identifying Jasmine's Distortions in Thinking

Before you look at your own thoughts, take a look at the way Jasmine thinks. Sometimes it's easier to learn to spot your own distorted thinking once you've observed it in a situation that doesn't hit so very close to home.

Jasmine is convinced that the blotches on her face are to blame for most things that have gone wrong in her life. The thoughts about her skin distort her self-image and make it difficult for her to be comfortable around men. She's 34 and firmly believes that she's not married and won't ever be because of these (actually relatively minor) blotches. Her friends often point out to her how intelligent, successful, and nice she is. They also tell her that the blotches aren't that noticeable, and that she looks just fine. But she doesn't believe them. Jasmine recently went out on a date. Here are some of the thoughts that ran through her mind during the evening:

> "The first thing he has noticed about me was my blotchy skin. He must have thought, 'Ugh, if I'd have known she looks like that, I wouldn't have come.' He kept staring at me all night long."

> "So what if I'm smart? All I really want is to look great! My life would be so much better if I were prettier."

> "He won't call me again. I'm so ugly; no one can ever fall in love with me. I'm a total failure."

Of course, every time she had these thoughts, Jasmine felt sad and hopeless about her future. You've probably already noticed that her thoughts contain some thinking errors. Why don't you see whether you can classify them? After you have made your attempt to find some errors in these thoughts, take a look at the errors that I found.

> **"The first thing he has noticed about me was my blotchy skin. He must have thought, 'Ugh, if I'd have known she looks like that, I wouldn't have come.' He kept staring at me all night long."**

Mind Reading

Jasmine makes assumptions about what her date might have noticed about her appearance, without having any clues about what is really going on in his head. This is a good example of the mind-reading error. She pays attention to what *she* considered to be wrong with her appearance, but she simply can't know what was running through his mind. He might have been thinking about their conversation, her beautiful hair, or the dinner. If he's like most people, he was actually thinking about himself or even his own appearance, but not Jasmine's skin. And even if he did notice some blotches, he might not care about them.

> **"So what if I'm smart? All I really want is to look great! My life would be so much better if I were prettier."**

Discounting the Positives, Magnification

At some point during the evening, Jasmine's date commented that she was pretty, smart, and fun to be around. Rather than appreciating this compliment, she put down all the wonderful things she had going for herself. She didn't care about being smart or that he enjoyed her company; all she focused on was the one thing she wished for: to look better. In this process, her blotches gained an all-powerful, life-changing status, and all her accomplishments and positive qualities were swept under the rug. In reality, it's not even clear whether and how her life would be different if she looked better. It's just as likely that her life would be exactly the same.

"He won't call me again. I'm so ugly; no one can ever fall in love with me. I'm a total failure."

Fortune Telling

Sad or horrific prophecies such as "He won't call me again" or "No one can ever fall in love with me" are usually a good clue to the fortune-telling error. Jasmine actually did not really have evidence for any of her negative predictions, and indeed, there was more evidence that he might call again, because he seemed to be enjoying himself.

Labeling, All-or-Nothing Thinking

This is a good example of how all-or-nothing thinking and labeling are contained in one thought. In fact, labeling is often a form of all-or-nothing thinking. Although Jasmine may have blotchy skin, she's not "ugly." Yes, she doesn't look perfect, but in reality, most people fall somewhere in between the two extremes of perfect and ugly on the beauty continuum. Also, just because her appearance isn't perfect doesn't mean that she's a complete "failure" as a person. Appearance is just one of many factors that people take into account when they choose other people as potential partners. Friendliness, intelligence, and trustworthiness are very important other qualities, too.

Magnification

In one thought, Jasmine went from having a few blotches on her skin to looking ugly. By doing this, she was magnifying the blotches, blowing them way out of proportion. People who aren't appearance-obsessed can disregard minor imperfections, because they don't think they are a big deal. Of course, they might not be thrilled about blotchy skin, pimples, or a receding hairline, but they don't really think they are ugly because of this. Since Jasmine overvalues the importance of these little blotches, she might believe that other people care much more about them—that the blotches reveal some personal flaw and are to blame for current or future unhappiness.

Emotional Reasoning

Jasmine assumes that she's ugly because she feels that way. In addition, she feels unlovable, even though she has absolutely no evidence for either one of the two.

Identifying Your Own Thinking Errors

Once you've finished recording your thoughts for a week, go back to the Thought Records and see whether the thoughts fit into one or maybe even several of the thinking error categories described. As soon as you find a particular error, write the error under the thought. After you have looked over all your Thought Records, check to see whether a particular error occurred more often than others. If so, this may be a very typical error for you.

Evaluating Your Thoughts

So far you've learned two important skills related to managing your thoughts: You've learned how to identify negative automatic thoughts and how to examine thinking errors. With the resulting skills and information as your foundation, you can learn to question—and, if necessary, modify—your unproductive thoughts. However, if you're like most people, you probably have many thoughts that are negative and contain thinking errors. So how do you select which thought(s) to work on?

The answer is simple: To learn the skills I describe, start with your *most recent* distressing thought. On some days you might have so many recent negative thoughts that it will be difficult to decide which ones to select for your exercises. If this is the case, write down all of the thoughts and rate them in terms of how frequent and distressing they are. Then start with the thought that is most responsible for your painful feelings. You can later work your way down to less distressing thoughts, and sometimes the need to work on those diminishes completely, if you've already dealt with the more bothersome thoughts.

If you have several recent distressing thoughts to choose from, keep the long-term goals you set in Chapter 4 in mind and start by working on the thoughts related to your most troubling problem area. Again, start with the thoughts that you gave the highest scores. After you've worked on those, consider others from the same problem area that are less important. Then you can move on to other problem areas. In addition to working on the thoughts that are currently distressing, focus on the thoughts you have collected over the course of the last week.

Question Yourself

If you've had a body image problem for a long time, you've also had negative thoughts about your appearance for a long time. You're probably so used to negative thoughts about your looks that you usually don't step back to ask yourself whether your thinking makes sense. But this is exactly what I'd like you to try next: I'd like you to try to take another look at your thoughts and evaluate them. A few years ago, Dr. Judith Beck came up with a number of questions to evaluate thoughts. I've changed these questions and added a few additional ones and have listed them in the box below. Not every question will be helpful for all of your negative thoughts. Many of these questions are particularly useful for certain thoughts, and some questions work better for others. Of course, there is no limit to the types of questions you could ask yourself, and over time, you'll probably come up with your own. For now, you just need to experiment to find out which questions may be helpful in evaluating a particular thought. I'm not saying that all of your thoughts are wrong. As a matter of fact, many of them con-

---

Questions to Help You Evaluate Your Negative Thoughts

Is this thought helpful right now? What are the advantages and disadvantages of this type of thinking? Is there a more advantageous point of view?

What is the evidence for my thought? What is the evidence against it? Which is more convincing?

So what if. . . ?

What is the worst that could happen if my fears came true? Could I live though it? Would it really change the big picture? Would I still care about it a few years down the road?

What is the best that could happen?

Is my thought logical? Is there another, perhaps more rational way of looking at that? Is there another explanation for. . . ?

Does . . . really mean that. . . ?

Am I really 100% certain that . . . , or is this just one out of many possibilities?

What would I tell a friend in this situation?

What would a friend say to me about this? What would my friend advise me to do?

What can I do now?

Adapted by permission of the publisher and author from Judith S. Beck, *Cognitive Therapy: Basics and Beyond* (Guilford Press, 1995).

---

tain some truth, and it's important for you to acknowledge this. But I'd like you to check out your thoughts to see whether a new or different perspective might be more appropriate or useful.

Fred, a shy 27-year-old pharmacist, had difficulty meeting women and was always the quiet one in a crowd. He was sure that anyone he talked to was staring at his "weak" chin, and these thoughts distorted his self-image and affected his self-worth. One day in the gym he noticed a woman his age and thought that he would like to ask her out, but several thoughts stood in his way:

"She won't like me because of my weak chin!" **(10)**

"I look so unmanly—what a loser!" **(10)**

"The only way I can be happy and successful is if I have surgery." **(6)**

"She'll never go out with me." **(5)**

"She may not like me after she gets to know me." **(3)**

"She might have a boyfriend, so she won't talk to me." **(3)**

As part of his treatment program, Fred first learned to rate the thoughts in terms of how distressing and frequent they were (ratings are in parentheses after the thought). Then he looked for the errors in his thinking. Next he used the questions above to evaluate his thoughts. He just tried out the questions in the list one by one. If the first question did not fit, he went to the next one. Next he just chose *the questions that best fit his thoughts.* As you can see, sometimes he had to modify the wording of the questions slightly so that they'd better apply to his thoughts. (In the following illustration I note only some of the questions that he ultimately chose to examine his thoughts.) Finally he put the answers to the question into words.

"She won't like me because of my weak chin!" (Mind Reading)

- *Is this thought helpful right now?* "No, it's not helpful at all."
- *What is the evidence for my thought that she'll notice my chin right away?* "Hmm, I don't really have any evidence, I guess."
- *What is the evidence against it?* "Well, nobody has ever really said anything awful about my chin, so it can't be that bad. Also, the chin isn't such a big part of my body or of who I am. She might notice other things first, like that I am tall, or that I like to dress in black, or that I have a good sense of humor."
- *Is the evidence for or against my thought more convincing?* "The evidence against it."
- *So what if . . . she doesn't like me because of my chin? What's the worst that could happen?* "It wouldn't be the end of the world, I guess. I'm not a robot, and it's normal to have a few imperfections. It's just part of being human; that's all. It's not like she'll start abusing me because I don't look like Superman. Also, I'm

not expecting her to be perfect either. If she didn't go out with me only because of the way my chin looks, she'd be a little superficial and probably wouldn't be a good date or girlfriend for me anyway."

• *What would my friends tell me?* "I guess my friends would say, 'The problem isn't how others see you; it's how you see yourself. That's what makes you anxious. . . . It's *you* who is worried about the chin, not her!' "

"I look so unmanly—what a loser!" (Labeling, All-or-Nothing Thinking)

• *Does having a less-than-perfect appearance equal being a loser?* "No, it doesn't. And even if my chin isn't as strong as I wish it were, who cares? I'm still a man and have many other masculine features. People actually have complimented me on my looks. The chin isn't such a big deal and doesn't make me a loser. I'm not going to make my self-worth depend on this one feature. There are so many things that matter more than my chin! I'm smart, athletic, and loyal to my friends."

"The only way I can be happy and successful is if I have plastic surgery." (All-or-Nothing Thinking, Fortune Telling, Discounting the Positives)

• *How helpful is this thought right now? What is the effect of this type of thinking?* "Well, this thought makes me feel sad, because it implies that I have to put my life on hold until I have surgery. It also puts down everything I've accomplished so far and makes it appear small and meaningless. So, I guess it's not a useful thought at all."

• *Is there another way of looking at that? Would my life really be different if my chin were more pronounced?* "Probably not. I'd still have the same job, the same friends, and the same hobbies. There are no laws that prevent people with smaller chins from being happy or having great accomplishments. So it's not really my chin that's the problem. It's the way I think about it that gets me in trouble. And that is something I'm just learning to change. I can have a good life even I don't look like a hunk. I just need to learn to accept myself."

"I can't talk to her. She won't go out with me anyway." (Fortune Telling)

• *What is the evidence that I can't talk to her? What is the evidence that I can?* "I don't have any evidence that I can't talk to her. All I have to do is come up with something to say. I could just comment that I like this gym and ask her if she's ever taken any of the classes."

• *What is the worst that could happen—and could I live through it?* "I doubt that she will start screaming or make some kind of a weird scene if I strike up a conversation. So I guess the worst would be that if I ask her she wouldn't go out with me. I wouldn't like it, but I could handle it."

• *Do I know for certain that she won't go out with me?* "No, I don't know for sure. I'm just afraid that she won't."

• *Is there any evidence that she may go out with me?* "Not really. She actually smiled when I looked at her earlier, so she might be interested in getting to know me. . . ."

As you can see, Fred started by questioning the thoughts that he rated most painful (in terms of distress and/or frequency). Then he worked his way down to less important thoughts. He did not even bother working on the thoughts that he rated only a 3, because they were not very disturbing. Writing down the answers to the questions helped Fred gain a new viewpoint on his thoughts. He noticed many things he had not considered before and realized that his original thoughts were not very logical or realistic.

Answer Your Negative Thoughts with a Rational Response

Fred's answers to the questions about his negative thoughts yielded a different perspective. He—and you—can now boil down those answers to a less detailed response to the negative thought. These "rational responses" have to be realistic and therefore credible. If Fred responded to the negative thought *She won't like me because of my weak chin!* with "She will be really impressed with me because I must be the best-looking guy she's ever seen!" his negative thought would probably win out, because he wouldn't believe his own statement about his appearance. For Fred a good rational response might have been "It's true that my chin is not as pronounced as I'd like it to be, but I don't have to look perfect for others to accept me." In developing this rational response, Fred took all the main points from the answers to the questions above into account.

As a next step I'd like you to try to come up with rational responses to your own negative thoughts. But first, let's see how Amy (on the facing page) applied her new skills to her automatic thoughts about going swimming. After recording the situation that made her feel bad and the negative thoughts associated with it, rating the thoughts in terms of related frequency and distress, and recording her feelings, she asked herself some questions pertaining to her most distressing thought ("If Jack is there, he'll find out what I really look like. He'll be so disappointed, he won't like me anymore") and answered them. The essence of these answers is captured in Amy's rational responses.

Now give it a shot and fill out your own Thought Record with any situation that has recently come up. But don't be disappointed if you don't really believe your rational response at first. After all, you might have been thinking irrational thoughts for a very long time. Consider this a learning process, like learning to use a stick shift. At first you are very aware of all the different steps you're taking. You have to think about hitting the brake, the gas pedal, and what to do with the clutch. Even changing the station on the radio while having to maneu-

Thought Record: Amy

Situation:

Thinking about going swimming.

Thoughts:

It will be really weird if I run into my classmates and I have no makeup on.   (5)
(Fortune Telling)

They'll think I look sick and pale.   (6)
(Mind Reading)

They'll stare at my small breasts.   (7)
(Fortune Telling)

If Jack is there, he'll find out what I really look like. He'll be so disappointed he won't like me anymore.   (9)
(Fortune Telling, Mind Reading, Magnification)

Feelings:

Anxious, frustrated

Questions:

What is the evidence for my prediction that Jack will be disappointed when he sees me in a bathing suit and without makeup?

   I don't really have any.

What is the evidence against it?

   I don't know how Jack feels about small breasts, but I am pretty sure that he's not really into makeup anyway. If he sees me in my bathing suit, he might notice my nice long legs, too. He has told me many times that he likes hanging out with me because I make him laugh. Recently he said he thought I was really sharp. Maybe these are the things he likes about me.

Rational response:

Just because I keep thinking about my breasts and skin doesn't mean that Jack does; he seems to like me because of other stuff.

Adapted by permission of the publisher and author from Judith S. Beck, *Cognitive Therapy: Basics and Beyond* (Guilford Press, © 1995).

Thought Record

Situation:

Thoughts:

Feelings:

Questions:

Rational response:

ver through traffic seems like a big risk. Every time you come to a hill, it feels like you'll roll backward (and you actually might roll back a little). But after some time you get more comfortable, and it doesn't feel like such a big production any longer. The same is true for learning how to develop rational responses. At first it may seem difficult or awkward, but over time, with continued practice, it will become second nature.

Try to fill out at least one Thought Record every day over the course of the next week. Make sure you address the thoughts that come up on a daily basis, but also keep going back to the goals you set in the previous chapter and pay particular attention to the thoughts that pertain to those goals. This may be difficult at first, but keep in mind that the more you practice, the more you'll improve. Briefly describe the situation, then write down the negative thoughts and rate each thought individually. Also write down the feelings caused by these thoughts. Next, try to see whether you can find the thinking errors, remembering that one thought can contain several thinking errors. Choose the most important thoughts and address them with the questions. The essence of the answers to these questions will help you formulate a rational response.

The cognitive techniques you've just learned—finding thinking errors, developing rational responses by disputing your thoughts, and completing thought records—are a very important part of this program. I recommend that you practice them for about 20–40 minutes per day over the course of the next week. These exercises will provide a basis for the exercises focused on behavioral change that follows in Chapters 6 and 7. Thereafter, you'll conduct behavioral exercises as well, and it might be sufficient to spend only 15–20 minutes per day on thought records (if, however, after 20 minutes you still feel that many thoughts cause you trouble, you should definitely keep going). Many of my patients incorporate the work on Thought Records permanently into their lives. However, as their symptoms improve, they start using the Thought Records (or at least the skills—identifying, evaluating, and modifying negative thoughts—they learned while using them) as needed.

Chapter 6

Getting Your Life Back with Exposure Exercises

In the previous chapter we took a closer look at the negative thoughts that underlie your appearance concerns. These thoughts and the related feelings of anxiety and embarrassment are the engines that drive your problem. But as you'll see, it's your avoidance behavior that keeps your engines running overtime. In this chapter, you'll focus on changing some of the behavior patterns that feed your appearance concerns. It's important to move on to the behavioral exercises 1 or 2 weeks after you've started working on your thoughts, even if the thoughts still cause you a lot of distress. As you'll realize over the next few weeks, this program works best once you learn to combine your work on thoughts and behavior changes flexibly, such as reducing avoidance behavior and rituals.

The first step in dealing with avoidance behavior is to understand how easily avoidance can steal away your enjoyment of life. When you feel anxious, self-conscious, or embarrassed (or expect to be), you want to get rid of these unpleasant feelings. This is only natural. To stop the bad feelings you avoid or escape from a situation by turning down invitations, skipping a class, staying home from a party, or not asking someone for a date. You probably also use more subtle avoidance strategies, such as turning your face away, avoiding certain body postures, using certain body parts or clothes to hide your perceived defect, evading eye contact, eluding or rejecting compliments, staying away from bright lights, combing your hair in a certain way, or applying lots of makeup. The

How to Stop Avoiding Compliments

It's common for people with appearance concerns to have a hard time with compliments, but this behavior isn't exactly like other subtle forms of avoidance. If you can't accept compliments, you might feel awkward when you receive them. Two common ways to avoid compliments are to shift the focus as soon as possible to the other person ("Oh, your hair looks terrific, too") and—worse—to disagree directly with the compliment ("I actually don't like the way my hair turned out"). If you have the tendency to reject compliments, you probably haven't thought about the impact this behavior has on others. They might feel rejected or feel like you're disregarding their opinion completely.

How can you work on your ability to accept compliments? First, you need to deal with any false assumptions you may have about what it means to accept a compliment. It doesn't mean you're vain, conceited, or arrogant. It simply means that you're willing to accept someone else's positive opinion of you. Why fight it? Also, keep in mind that's it's OK to feel good about yourself. Of course, to have the skill of accepting compliments, you need to know what to say and do in response to a compliment. The easiest response is simply to make eye contact, smile, and say "Thank you." After you become more skilled with this simple response, you may next want to try to have a brief conversation about the compliment. Try agreeing with the person and adding your opinion ("Yes, I really like this blouse on me, too. I think the color of this skirt is really nice").

Remember that work on accepting compliments should be a regular part of your exposure program. It can have some surprisingly powerful effects on changing the way you view yourself in social situations. Make sure to practice regularly.

immediate payoff of avoidance is relief from fears of embarrassment or humiliation related to your appearance concerns.

But you have to keep in mind that this relief comes at a cost. With avoidance, you won't have a chance to see how things would have turned out had you not hidden. Maybe it would have been just fine. But since you were avoiding, you'll never know. In short, avoidance increases your fears by reducing your chances to learn that your fears aren't accurate. Avoidance also saps your confidence that you can handle the situation without hiding or escaping next time it comes up.

Think of a person who, fearing a nuclear missile attack, locks herself in a bomb shelter. Once in the underground shelter, she loses contact with the world, and she can't tell whether the missile attack has begun. She's lonely, the shelter is dark, and she misses the fresh food she used to enjoy. She'd like to leave the shelter and return to life, but she just feels too unsafe. She fears that opening the door will expose her to deadly radiation. So she stays locked inside, never knowing whether her fears are exaggerated, never getting the chance to see whether there's been an attack. She stays in the shelter for many years. When she finally gets very old and feels she's going to die soon, she decides to climb up the stairs. She opens the shelter, and with one look around she realizes that *nothing* had happened. There's no radiation, and there was no attack.

With respect to your appearance concerns, avoidance is like a bomb shelter, where you try to hide from fears of rejection, criticism, and humiliation. Over time, it feels like staying in the shelter is the only safe way to go on with life. But you need to evaluate the cost of your avoidance relative to your desire to be involved in life. In this chapter, I'll ask you to test whether your fears are realistic and suggest that we venture into the world outside the shelter of your current avoidance patterns. I'll also encourage you to invest some anxiety into the possibility that it's safe to come out of hiding. If you dare to come out of the shelter of avoidance, you, too, will discover that (other than perhaps getting a little anxious at first) *nothing* bad will happen. In this chapter I'll show you that you can improve your life when you take a stand against the deception of avoidance.

Thinking about Leaving the Shelter: What Is the Goal?

Of course, anyone who works on overcoming avoidance would like to do so without experiencing anxiety. This is difficult. Can you imagine leaving a bomb shelter after several years without feeling anxious when cracking open the door, venturing up the stairs, or stepping out into the sunlight? Anxiety is a normal part of reducing avoidance. Nonetheless, you'll learn to minimize your anxiety as you try to overcome your appearance concerns.

The process of overcoming fears and avoidance by doing is called *exposure*. In exposure practice you'll face situations that make you anxious. Now you probably think, "No way! Are you crazy? I'd never do that! There's a reason I avoid all this! I'd be much too scared!" Don't worry, I'm not planning on overwhelming you. We'll go step-by-step to help you get comfortable gradually with the situations you still fear. And we'll go only as fast as you are able to go.

Let me give you an example of the very first patient I treated with exposure. Neysa was afraid of heights. First she practiced standing on a second-floor balcony. Initially she was quite anxious that she might fall down, and she held on to the railing with white knuckles. But she didn't give up, and after about half an hour, she felt a lot more comfortable. She was ready to move on. So she proceeded to the third floor, fourth floor, fifth floor, and so on. She'd learn from her own experience that although she initially *felt* unsafe, she'd never fall down or faint. She learned that it was actually safe to be on the balcony. With repeated practice, venturing out on higher balconies no longer felt frightening to her. After she finally leaned over the railing of a 20th-floor balcony, the ones on the lower floors seemed like a piece of cake. "I feel so good about what I've accomplished," she said. "I never thought I'd be able to do that."

Exposure practice also plays an important role in helping you deal with your appearance concerns. One important part of your exposure practice is learning the difference between the way situations *feel* and how they actually *are*. The goal is to tolerate your negative thoughts and feelings long enough to experience the fact that a feared situation is actually safe. Exposure is a central part of the treatment of anxiety problems and has been shown to be a powerful technique in many research studies. I use it with my patients on a daily basis, and I'm often amazed to see that after only a few sessions, patients are able to do things they never thought they'd be able to handle. As I said, we make sure that your exposure practices aren't overwhelming by starting with easier ones and working our way up to harder ones. Also, the cognitive skills from Chapter 5 will help you reduce the anxiety you may feel, and over time, you'll be able to handle more challenging situations than you can probably imagine right now.

"How Can I Go Out If I Think People Find Me Hideous?"

The purpose of exposure is to examine whether you can have a good social life or meet other personal goals despite your appearance concerns. Janet is concerned about a few small acne scars and practically invisible facial hair. By objective standards, she is attractive and successful, and she'd like to be in a relationship, but she turns down dates because she doesn't want anyone to get a close look at her face. If we examine Janet's thoughts, it's obvious that others don't find her hideous, as she claims, because if that were true, she probably wouldn't even be asked out. She has evidence that others find her attractive, but she pays attention only to her negative beliefs. Janet would probably have successful relationships if she'd confront her fears and go on those dates. But she never puts her assumptions that she'll be rejected to the test.

In exposure practice you learn to face your fears. You resume activities that you might have been avoiding for a long time. If you're ready to jump right in and do really difficult exposures, then that's great. But most likely, you'll go a little slower, step-by-step. Your successful experiences will reduce your anxiety and change your thoughts. But you have to dare to test your negative assumptions about what will happen when you stop avoiding. I'll also show you that you can have a fulfilling social life even if you think that your appearance is not perfect.

"But I've *Tried* to Get On with My Life—It Doesn't Work"

Often my patients tell me that they have already tried to stay in feared situations, before they started this program, but they're still terrified. What they don't realize is that their efforts need to be systematic to lead to improvement. They need to stay in the situation long enough to get comfortable. They need to work on the negative thinking that feeds their anxiety. Without those measures, efforts at exposure are haphazard and don't build toward improvement.

Also keep in mind that even subtle avoidance behaviors can keep fears alive. Janet has a habit of averting her face to the side and downward, so that her hair falls against her cheeks, the area of her greatest appearance concerns. Janet doesn't know that by always hiding her cheeks when talking to others, she prevents herself from having the experience that others will actually continue to like her even after having seen her "flaws."

How Does Exposure Work?

Exposure will help you get comfortable with reentering avoided situations. After a while, you'll get used to them, or "habituate," as psychologists call it. I know that you'll be anxious when you first enter a situation you normally avoid. That's why it's important that you stay in the situation long enough to have a chance to bring your anxiety down. A well-arranged exposure practice also gives you the chance to compare your fears to your real-life experiences. During this practice, it'll be important for you to test whether your feared outcomes actually occur. If your experiences are successful and your feared outcomes don't come true, your fears will fade with repeated practice. You'll probably have to repeat the exposures (and learning experiences) several times, until you become comfortable in the situation.

Why Is Repeated Practice Helpful?

If you enter situations you normally avoid over and over again, and nothing bad happens, over time you learn that the situations are actually safe. It might be easier to understand what I mean if you think of a thriller or some other scary movie. The first time you see it, you may find it frightening. But if you watch the movie over and over again, it loses its ability to scare you. You become used to it. You know what's about to happen, and you become comfortable (or even bored) seeing it.

This is the reason for repeated exposure practice. It's likely that you'll have anxiety the first several times you try exposure practices, but eventually your anxiety will decrease. The aim is to start small and build confidence as you learn to get more comfortable with less frightening situations and events before trying really difficult exposures.

"How Much Time Should I Invest in My Program?"

In Chapter 5, I asked you to work on your negative thoughts for at least 20 minutes every day. I'd also like you to engage in exposure to avoided situations every day. From this point forward, you want to invest at least 45–60 minutes per day in your program. About half of this time should be spent doing Thought Records, and the other half, on practicing exposure. You can always do more, if you like. Remember, the more time you spend doing these exercises, the faster you will improve.

Managing Your Anxiety during Exposure

As I mentioned, we'll keep your anxiety at a manageable level by taking a gradual approach, working our way up a hierarchy, ranging from situations that are only somewhat anxiety provoking to more challenging ones, but only as you're ready to do so. If you do get anxious during an exposure, the most important thing to remember is that the feeling won't last forever. Also keep in mind that having anxiety doesn't mean that your negative thoughts are going to come true. In Chapter 5 you learned about emotional reasoning, the belief that any thought that *feels* true *is* true. You can now see that with emotional reasoning it'll always feel too unsafe to leave the bomb shelter of avoidance. Anxiety is a natural part of opening the door, and it will feel like there's dangerous radiation outside. If you "believe" this feeling, you may never allow yourself to leave the shelter. So what is the alternative? You must fully participate in life *despite* feeling somewhat anxious.

If you're really anxious about practicing a certain exposure, try to determine the thoughts that pertain to the exposure situation. If you cannot predict what you might think, close your eyes and try to picture yourself in the actual situation. Once you've identified some negative thoughts, work on them with a Thought Record, developing a rational response ahead of time. Then write down the rational response and review it frequently. (You might want to write it on a little index card, so you can carry it with you and look at it when you need it.)

Nevertheless, although the cognitive strategies can help quite a bit, keep in mind that they're not a miracle cure, and even if you use your cognitive skills well, most likely some anxiety will remain. For many people, the moments right before the exposure and the early part of the exposure are the most anxiety provoking. This is anxiety in anticipation of facing your fears. If you can hang in there, you'll see that the anxiety will come down. And remember that it's OK to have some anxiety during this program; you are investing this anxiety in a better future.

Preparing for Your Exposure Practices

The first step in thinking about exposure is organizing your avoidance patterns into a list, then ordering the list from less difficult to more difficult exposures. Begin by reviewing the Long-Term Goals Worksheet for your most important major problem area in Chapter 4, paying particular attention to the section "Related avoidance behavior." The long-term goals are usually very broad and should guide the general direction you take in treatment. Next, fill out the Distress-Provoking Situations Worksheet on page 114 and write down the specific situations that you are avoiding or enduring with discomfort, and that pertain to your most important major problem area. Reviewing your answers to the assessment, Situations You Are Likely to Avoid or Endure with Discomfort (pp. 63–64), due to body image concerns will provide you with crucial background information on your problem. Try to be as specific as you can when writing down the situations that bother you.

Consider the example of Ada from Chapter 4. One of her long-term goals was to decrease avoidance behavior in social situations where family, friends, and coworkers were present. This long-term goal was not very specific, so she next thought of specific situations in which she was actually having trouble, and wrote down the situations, such as going to church and sitting in the front row, going to church and sitting in the last row, shaking hands with other parishioners after church, and so forth.

Now it's your turn. Write down 10–15 situations that pertain to your long-term goals and that you avoid because you feel distressed, ashamed, or anxious about your appearance. Remember that avoidance behaviors can be subtle (for example, covering your perceived flaw with your body position or hair, avoiding eye contact, avoiding light that would hit your presumed defect in a certain way). Be honest with yourself and look at your behavior squarely, so that you can spot avoidance.

Sometimes people have a hard time thinking of situations they need to work on. Maybe the following examples of situations my patients have worked on will give you some ideas.

- Going to a family gathering or party; getting a haircut; going to church, temple, mosque
- Sitting across from someone, sitting in the front row
- Going on a date
- Interacting with someone who looks good in areas where you feel you are lacking (for example, if you think you're too short, talk to someone who is really tall)

- Having a checkup at your doctor's office, where you have to reveal body part(s) of concern
- Engaging in an activity that makes it impossible to hide your perceived flaws (for example, going swimming, which messes up your hair, or going to a sauna, where you can't wear clothing or makeup to hide your flaws)
- Getting your picture taken
- Leaving the house and going for a short walk without makeup, without a hat, without having your hair styled, and without sunglasses
- Having close physical contact (for example, allowing someone to touch a flaw or look at it from a short distance)
- Making eye contact with a stranger
- Sitting close to a person (and exposing the body part of concern)
- Sitting/standing under a bright light, being outside on a sunny day and not avoiding the bright daylight
- Showing your flaws (for example, smiling to expose crooked teeth, wrinkles; wearing clothing that doesn't cover your imperfections, such as a tank top that reveals freckles on your arms)
- Keeping the light on when you undress in front of your partner and engage in sexual positions that expose your flaws
- Going to places where appearance is emphasized (for example, a gym with mirrors on the wall, a singles gathering, a dressy occasion, expensive stores, or makeup counters)

I'm sure that many situations make you anxious, but put on your list only those related to the goals you actually want to reach in this program. Because we'll select your short-term goals from this list, also be sure to write down only situations that can be arranged in future exposure practices (for example, it may be difficult for you to arrange an appearance on stage or on TV). The more specific you can be with your situations, the better. Instead of "going out with friends," write "going to the mall with John and Beverly." After you've written down some situations, you need to rate the intensity of your distress. I think it's easiest to use a scale ranging from 0 to 100. A rating of 0 means that the situation is not distressing for you at all. A rating of 100 means the situation is as distressing as you can imagine. If you think the situation is only mildly uncomfortable, rate it as a 10 or 20. If you think the situation causes you moderate distress, rate it at about 50. If you believe that the situation would make you highly distressed, rate it as 70–80.

Next, examine whether you always avoid distressing situations. Please rate each situation according to the degree to which you avoid it. In the Distress-Provoking Worksheet, rate how often you avoid each situation, again using a scale of 0–100. Zero means you never avoid this situation, 50 means you avoid it about 50% of the time, 100 means you always avoid it. Also use the percentages in between; for example, if you sometimes avoid it, give it a 10 or 20, and if you often avoid it, give it a 75 or 80.

Distress-Provoking Situations Worksheet

Distress-provoking situations	Degree of distress (1–100)	Degree to which I avoid (1–100)
1.		
2.		
3.		
4.		
5.		
6.		
7.		
8.		
9.		
10.		
11.		
12.		
13.		
14.		
15.		

Exposure Worksheet

My exposure situation (be specific):

What aspect of the situation causes me the most distress?

What subtle ways of avoiding do I need to watch out for?

Preparing my thoughts:

Negative thoughts/predictions   Alternative thoughts

Goals for the exposure—How will I know I did well? (objective criteria):

1.

2.

3.

(continued)

Exposure Worksheet (continued)

Distress rating:
Beginning:
Middle:
End:

Evaluating my efforts:
Did I reach my goal(s)?

Did my negative thoughts/predictions come true?

What did I learn?

How will I reward myself?

Go for It: Conducting Your First Exposure

Choosing a Situation to Work On in Exposure Practice

Now that you've identified situations that you avoid, you'll need to pick the first situation you want to work on in exposure practice. I suggest you start with a situation in which you have moderate distress and avoidance, with a rating near 40 or 50. Go ahead, select one situation, then fill in the first row on the Exposure Worksheet. Describe which characteristics of the situation are most bothersome to you. Also write on your worksheet whether there are any subtle avoidance behaviors you need to watch out for.

To give you an idea of what we're trying to accomplish, take a look at John's Exposure Worksheet. John, an athletic 22-year-old, thinks he's not muscular enough, particularly that his thighs are "too thin" and he therefore looks "unmanly" or like a "sissy." Because of these concerns he avoids going to the beach or wearing a bathing suit. The idea of going to the beach in a swimsuit causes him moderate (45) distress. What bothers him most about being on the beach is talking to others while standing. Accordingly, he'd complete the first section of his Exposure Worksheet as follows:

My exposure situation (be specific):
Going to the beach for 1 hour on Saturday with Chuck, Paul, and Ed

What aspect of the situation causes me the most distress?
Standing on the sand, talking with friends

What subtle ways of avoiding do I need to watch out for?
Lying on my towel instead of standing up

Addressing Your Negative Thinking

Think of your exposure practice as an experiment that will allow you to prove or disprove some of your more frightening thoughts. After you have selected the situation you'd like to work on, anticipate the negative thoughts that may pop up, so you can counter them ahead of time to make the exposure much easier. Picture yourself in the selected situation. Imagine the whole scene. What kinds of thoughts run through your mind as you think about your exposure exercise? Try to discover as many thoughts as you can. Don't edit your thoughts or pretty them up. Write them on the Exposure Worksheet in the space for negative thoughts. Now apply the cognitive techniques you learned in Chapter 4. Start by evaluating whether you made any thinking errors and whether any other alternative thoughts may be more useful or more valid. You can use the questions from Chapter 4 that help you formulate a rational response. Remember, if you can change the negative thoughts about the situations that scare you, your discomfort will go down. This work on your thoughts will help you with your exposure exercises, because it ensures that your negative thoughts and feelings won't catch you off guard. You expected them, and now you have a strategy to cope with them.

Using this method, John generated the following alternative thoughts for his Exposure Worksheet.

Preparing my thoughts:

Negative thoughts/predictions	Alternative thoughts
Everyone will stare at my legs	*(All-or-Nothing Thinking). Just because I'm concerned about my legs doesn't mean everyone else is. My friends will be more interested in women than my legs.*
My legs are hideously thin	*(Labeling). Nobody has ever said anything negative about my legs. Plus, it's OK if my legs aren't perfect. I don't judge others on the basis of the shape of their legs either.*

Deciding on Specific, Achievable, and Objective Goals

It is important to set *specific* goals before you start an exposure, so that you can tell in the end whether you've been successful. If your goals weren't specific, it's just too easy to discount the whole exercise because you got anxious or it didn't go perfectly in some other way. Also, after you're done with the exercise, knowing that you reached a specific goal will give you a feeling of accomplishment. And knowing which goals caused you difficulty will give you an idea of what to work on in the future. A common mistake in early exposure work is to have unrealistic or perfectionistic goals.

Let's assume, for example, that John set goals of going to the beach, feeling comfortable (not anxious), and having no one look at his legs. These goals are unrealistic for an initial exposure. John based the success of his practice on his *feelings* (no anxiety). However, we already know that he'll probably feel anxious;

this is why he's applying this treatment program in the first place. So the goal of not getting anxious didn't meet the criterion of being achievable at this point. Of course, one of his long-term aims for therapy is to feel better in situations that make him anxious right now. And all of the techniques we have discussed so far will help him move in this direction. But aiming for not being anxious as the goal of a specific exercise is not a good idea. For now, we are working directly on changing behaviors and thoughts. As you'll recall from previous chapters, thoughts, feelings, and behaviors are closely related; therefore, John's negative feelings will also change eventually. But this usually takes a little more time. Any goal that involves feelings (for example, not feeling anxious, feeling self-confident) is also problematic because it is not *objective*. Others would have a hard time evaluating accurately how anxious he is; usually, only John himself would be able to tell.

John also made the successful outcome of his exercise dependent on what *others* do (look at his legs or not). But it is actually very tricky to make the behavior (or feelings) of others part of your goals, because you have only very limited control over what they do or feel. Instead, it would be much better for John to set specific goals that have to do with his *own behavior*. Here are the objective and achievable goals John finally decided on:

Goals for the exposure—How will I know I did well? (objective criteria):

1. Stay at the beach for 1 hour even if I get anxious.
2. Stand up for at least part of the time (at least 10 minutes).

Evaluating and Rewarding Your Efforts

After you have finished the exposure, now matter how well it went, congratulate yourself for having tried it. Then complete the Exposure Worksheet. The last spaces are reserved for the evaluation of your efforts. Because exposure exercises can be powerful learning experiences, it's important to put your results in writing.

Rating Your Distress

After each exposure it's important to evaluate your distress using the 0–100 scale. How distressed were you right before you started? Did your distress rise or fall during the exposure practice? Did you end up being more comfortable at the end than at the beginning of the exposure? The ratings can also help you track your progress over the course of this program. Next time you work on the same situation, you'll probably see that the rating at the beginning of the exposure is lower than the rating you started with the last time. This is exactly what happened to John:

Distress rating:
Beginning: 85
Middle: 60
End: 35

Reviewing Whether You Reached Your Goal(s)

Next, look back at your specific goal(s) and decide whether you met them. However, watch out for the unhelpful thought patterns introduced in Chapter 5 and be careful not to fall into the traps of selectively attending to the things that went wrong during the exposures or discounting the positive aspects of your practice. Many of the people I've worked with over the years have paid too much attention to little imperfections in the exposure and were therefore likely to miss all the wonderful things they did correctly. For example, after completing his exposure practice, I asked John how it went. He looked a bit discouraged and said: "It didn't go very well. I was really nervous. Especially when I first went there." I pointed out that "not getting nervous" was not on the list of goals he'd decided on prior to practicing exposure. So we took a look at the goals he'd actually set: Stay at the beach for 1 hour even if I get anxious; stand up for at least part of the time (at least 10 minutes). It turned out that he'd met both goals. In fact, he'd done even better than expected, because he was able to stay on the beach for 3 hours, and he stood up talking to his friends for altogether about half an hour. So reviewing whether he met the goals he set before he did the exposure helped John see that he had been successful.

Always make sure you review the specific goals you were trying to accomplish. Then write down if you were successful! Here is what John wrote after our discussion:

Did I reach my goal(s)? Yes. I even did more than I'd planned.

But what if you have trouble and don't meet an exposure goal? Don't be surprised if exposures don't always go as well as you'd hoped. Remember that over the course of the program you'll have to repeat the exercises several times before you really conquer your fears. If you have difficulty with one particular exposure exercise, break it down into smaller, more manageable steps. For example, if you normally try to hide your pale skin by covering it with makeup and can spend only a few minutes outside your own home without makeup at first, that's OK. In future exposures you can increase your time by adding on more minutes.

Reviewing Your Thoughts

Always record, on copies of the Exposure Worksheet, what actually happened in the situation and whether your negative thoughts or predictions came true.

You'll probably see that, most of the time, the negative predictions you made prior to your exercise were wrong. If any unexpected negative thoughts came up, write them down on a Thought Record, evaluate them, and, if appropriate, try to come up with alternative thoughts and review this Thought Record prior to your next exposure. Here is what John wrote about his predictions and his learning experience during this exposure practice:

> *Did my negative thoughts/predictions come true?* No they didn't. I really don't think that anyone cared about my legs.
>
> *What did I learn?* My legs are probably not as noticeable as I thought they were.

Rewarding Yourself

Finally, don't forget to reward yourself for your efforts. You made a first attempt at facing your fears, and that's just great. You can reward yourself by taking time off to do a favorite activity, watch a favorite TV show, or buy something you've been wanting for a long time. Here's how John rewarded himself:

> *How will I reward myself?* Watch *Star Trek* tonight.

Should I Tell Anyone about My Exposure Practices?

If you have a supportive friend or family member, ask whether he or she would like to help you practice. Be sure to pick someone (or several people) you trust and who understands your problem. Talk to your support team about your avoided situations and discuss your goals. You may even schedule when they work with you. A supportive person might encourage you to hang in there when the going gets tough, and this will make distressing situations easier to bear.

Tom's First Exposure

Tom, a 25-year-old software programmer, works in a small firm. He does his job well and is thought to be a nice guy by his friends and coworkers. However, Tom doesn't like being around people, especially if he doesn't know them very well. He's an expert in inventing excuses about why he cannot go to parties or other social gatherings. He's convinced that his teeth are yellow and crooked, and that his hair is too thin. He doesn't like to smile because it exposes his teeth. In addition, he avoids showing his teeth by putting his hands in front of his mouth when he speaks. He never has his picture taken and avoids looking at his old photographs. Tom's most distressing major problem area is his hair, because he's concerned that it's thinning. His most important long-term goal is not to avoid situations that make him self-conscious about his hair. For example, Tom avoids haircuts, because he never likes their results. In addition, on days when he feels particularly bad about his hair, he wears hats. Tom has never told his girlfriend about his "defects," because he's worried that this would cause her to notice them even more than she does now.

Tom started his program by telling his girlfriend Jenny about his problem. Although she couldn't see that he was getting bald and didn't really think his crooked teeth looked so bad, much to his surprise, she was very supportive and even suggested that she help him work on his problem. After listing the situations that Tom avoided, they started by setting goals mainly related to his hair. Then they began looking for an appropriate situation for Tom's first exposure practice.

He picked a situation that caused him moderate distress for his first exposure (see Exposure Worksheet on the facing page).

As you can see, Tom set a very specific goal and successfully used the cognitive techniques described in Chapter 5. Tom's distress rating began at 43. In the middle, his distress increased a little, because he thought that the hairdresser was reacting negatively to his hair. But once he remembered the rational response he had developed ahead of time, his anxiety decreased again. After 30 minutes, his distress rating had already dropped to 20. This is fairly typical. However, sometimes you may have a tough day and feel like you aren't moving forward at all. In these situations, try to remember that learning a new skill doesn't happen overnight. Don't be discouraged if on some days you struggle or make no progress at all, because on other days, your improvement will be greater.

How Do You Practice Exposure over Time?

In the previous section, you learned how to design your first exposure practice. But, of course, if you're like most of the people I've worked with, many different situations bother you. So how do you decide the order in which you should select them for exposure practice? As we discussed, you should start with an exposure that focuses on avoidance behavior that's related to the major problem area that causes you the most distress. Your first exposure situation should cause you only moderate distress. Work on it every day, until the distress has decreased substantially (e.g., to a distress rating of 25 or lower) and until you don't avoid the situation any longer. It's probably a good idea to repeat the exposure a couple of times even if your distress rating is at 25 or lower, to be sure that you've really mastered a specific situation. Initially you'll work on one situation only; however, as soon as you've become a little more comfortable with the situation, you should add more situations. If you have many beauty rituals as well, exposure practice alone is not enough, and you'll need to incorporate response prevention

Exposure Worksheet: Tom

My exposure situation (be specific):
Get hair shampooed and cut tomorrow afternoon at 3 (tomorrow is Tuesday, and it won't be so crowded).

What aspect of the situation causes me the most distress?
Seeing myself in the mirror.

What subtle ways of avoiding do I need to watch out for?
Avoiding eye contact with my hairdresser and avoiding looking in the mirror

Preparing my thoughts:

Negative thoughts/predictions	Alternative thoughts
My hairdresser will be grossed out by my thin hair.	*It doesn't help me if I try to read minds. There's no evidence that she'll be grossed out by my hair. In fact, last time I was there, she was actually really nice to me.*

Goals for the exposure—How will I know I did well? (objective criteria):
Getting my hair cut is the goal; it's OK if I feel anxious. I'll also look in the mirror at least three times and make eye contact three times.

Distress rating:
Beginning: 43
Middle: 50
Ending: 20

Evaluating my efforts:
Did I reach my goal(s)?
I reached my goals. I got my hair cut, and I looked at her and in the mirror three times.

Did my negative thoughts/predictions come true?
It actually went better than I thought it would. She didn't seem to be grossed out. Initially I was pretty self-conscious, but when I stopped reading her mind and started chatting about my job, I felt better. I think I'm starting to make progress.

What did I learn?
Once I get through the initial anxiety, it gets easier. People seem to like me and respect me as I am.

How will I reward myself?
Go to see movie with Jenny tonight.

into your exercises. I'll show you how to do this in Chapter 7. Ultimately you want to be sure that you work on exposure (and, later, exposure and response prevention) for at least 45–60 minutes per day. Thus, for most people that means working on several situations over the course of 1 week (and sometimes even over the course of 1 day), especially if these exposures are tied to events that do not necessarily occur every day (for example, going to a holiday party or other dressy occasion), or if the individual exposures are brief (for example, asking a stranger a question while exposing the perceived defect). Over the course of the next few weeks, you'll work your way up your distressing situations hierarchy step-by-step, so that your most feared situations are completed in the latter part of the program. Continue with the program until you have successfully confronted even the most difficult situations on your list.

Tom, the software programmer with the hair and teeth concerns described earlier, worked his way up his distressing situations hierarchy over 2 months. Take a look at what kind of exposure he practiced at various stages of his program. Please note that his first week of exposure practice corresponds to the fourth week of the overall BDD program. (It took him 1 week to learn about BDD, complete the initial assessments, and set treatment goals; then he spent 2 weeks on identifying and changing his negative thoughts.)

Exposures Tom Conducted during the First Week of Exposure Practice

- Got my hair shampooed and cut on a Tuesday
- Stopped wearing hats, no matter where I went (daily)

Exposures Tom Conducted during the Second Week of Exposure Practice

- No longer wore hats
- Looked at old pictures for 30 minutes (daily, until the distress rating decreased to 25)
- Showed old pictures to my girlfriend for 1 hour

Exposures Tom Conducted during the Fourth Week of Exposure Practice

- No longer wore hats
- Showed old pictures to other friends for 1 hour
- Had my pictures taken by my girlfriend (for about 30 minutes)
- Had my picture taken in a photo studio
- Appeared in a family video

- Went to a family event and stayed for at least 2 hours, without covering my teeth; tried to smile at least five times
- Went to social gathering where I knew few people and stayed for 1 hour without covering my teeth; tried to smile at least 10 times

Exposures Tom Conducted during the Final Weeks of Exposure Practice

- No longer wore hats
- Continued to arrange or attend social events (at least two per week; made sure I smiled frequently)
- Continued to have pictures and videos taken, and showed photographs whenever the opportunity presented itself
- Got my hair cut on a Saturday (when it's very crowded)
- Went to the grocery store with wet hair and stayed for 30 minutes (three times a week) [Wet hair was particularly difficult for Tom, because he felt that his hair looked really thin when it was wet.]
- Walked around on the street with wet hair twice a week

Because Tom had hardly any appearance rituals, his treatment plan focused predominantly on exposure. (Because most people with body image concerns engage in avoidance behavior and rituals, in the next chapter, I'll show you another patient's treatment plan, which incorporates both exposure and response prevention.) Initially Tom worked on only one major body area, but over time he started adding more exposures that pertained to the same body area, as well as exposures related to goals regarding different body areas. This way he ensured that he practiced for at least 45–60 minutes every day. In addition to working on those exposures, Tom was very active in completing Thought Records daily. This increased the effectiveness of the exposure exercises. You might have noticed that, in addition to exposure to avoided situations, he stopped hiding the body parts he was concerned about (he no longer used a hat to hide his hair, and he stopped using his body position, particularly his hands, to hide his teeth). By working on those exposures, Tom made an important discovery. He had faced many threatening situations without hiding, and still nothing bad had happened. Nobody screamed, laughed, or treated him badly. Learning from experience that people accepted him as he really was helped him feel more self-confident. Tom reassessed himself frequently over the course of his program to ensure that he was on track with respect to completing his short- and long-term goals. After 12 weeks, he had reached all his long-term goals. Tom told me that he now enjoyed social events he used to dread. He also described his treatment experience as follows: "I feel free. No more hiding, no more excuses, no more fear of discovery. I can accept myself much better now. People got to know the true me over the course of this program, and it was nice to see that they like me just as much."

How Should You Evaluate Your Progress?

Just like Tom, you need to evaluate your progress frequently. You know that you've successfully completed a particular exposure if you got your distress rating reliably down to 25 or lower and you no longer avoid the specific situation. In other words, you can easily determine how you're doing with respect to reaching short-term goals by monitoring your daily distress ratings on the Exposure Worksheet. About once a month you should also retake the assessment from Chapter 4, Situations You Are Likely to Avoid or Endure with Discomfort (pp. 63–64) due to body image concerns. Redoing this assessment will give you a good idea of where you stand with respect to your long-term goals as well.

What's Next?

Now, if you haven't started yet, it's time to get to work. Take one of your problems listed in the Distress-Provoking Situations Worksheet, convert it into a specific goal, and write it on the Exposure Worksheet. If you have a support person, he or she should assist you in choosing your goals. Correct any negative thoughts or predictions you might have about the situations you want to conquer. I strongly recommend that you save your Exposure Worksheets after you're done with a particular exercise; they'll help you keep track of your process. Look back at these pages often, because they can help you with the particular goals on which you're working.

Chapter 7

Freeing Yourself
from Rituals with Response
Prevention Exercises

In Chapter 6, we talked about reducing your avoidance behavior with a powerful technique called *exposure practice*. Exposure helps you to go back and experience situations that you might have been avoiding or that make you very uncomfortable. But avoidance and rituals are the twin engines that keep your body image problem going over time, and exposure will have only a limited effect on your beauty rituals. Rituals make you feel better temporarily but in the long run, they actually feed your embarrassment and anxiety.

Rituals related to appearance concerns, such as body or mirror checking, reassurance seeking, excessive grooming or appearance fixing, excessive shopping or exercising, and skin picking, may take from a few minutes to several hours each day. Very time-consuming rituals can take the place of healthier behaviors, such as working or spending time with family or friends. So just like avoidance, rituals steal the fun from your life!

As with avoidance behaviors, engaging in rituals prevents you from seeing that things would have turned out just fine without the rituals, and from coming up with healthier coping strategies for managing your fears. For example, if you always ritualize, you're less likely to test your new cognitive strategies. Therefore, to fully reduce appearance concerns, you'll also have to stop the rituals in which you engage.

Occasionally I come across patients who have very few, if any, rituals. These people are treated predominantly with the cognitive techniques and exposure described in previous chapters. But most people with body image concerns have at least a couple of appearance-related rituals. Therefore, it's very important that you combine the ritual prevention techniques described in this chapter with the strategies described in Chapters 5 and 6. If you engage in avoidance behaviors, as well as appearance rituals, move on to ritual prevention within a few days after starting exposure. Just practice exposure by itself, long enough to get a sense of how it works, then add on the technique described in this chapter, which therapists call *response prevention*, meaning that you prevent yourself from responding to anxiety or discomfort with the usual rituals. The reason you need to add response prevention to your program soon after starting exposure is that you may not habituate to a situation during exposure practice if you are still ritualizing.

How Does Response Prevention Work?

Response prevention works just like exposure. When you stop or decrease your rituals, most likely you'll feel distressed at first. You must let your feelings calm down on their own, without ritualizing, or you won't weaken the urges to engage in unhealthy appearance behaviors. If you ritualize, your exposure exercise won't be helpful, because you won't have the opportunity to find out that the situation would have turned out just fine without ritualizing. Eventually you'll get used to handling situations without ritualizing. You'll weaken the mental connection between your rituals and temporarily feeling good and, with time, patience, and determination, reduce the urge to perform the rituals.

Preparing for Response Prevention

Choosing the Ritual(s) You Want to Decrease

If, like most people with body image concerns, you have multiple rituals, the first step in reducing your rituals is to choose the ones you want to decrease. The first criterion for selection is the relevance to your long-term goals; the second criterion is the distress that interrupting the ritual will cause. Start by reviewing the long-term goals you want to reach. In Chapter 6, you learned to decrease avoidance behaviors in situations associated with these long-term goals. If there are rituals associated with the exposure exercises you've conducted so far, target them first. Write down all the rituals associated with your first exposure and rate on a scale of 0–100 the distress they'd cause if they were interrupted and the frequency/time spent ritualizing.

If your main problem is ritualizing, and you didn't really conduct exposures after reading Chapter 6 because you don't avoid many situations, you'll start ritual prevention by rating rituals that occur in a situation associated with your first major problem area. Those trigger situations might be, for example, getting ready to leave the house, meeting friends, going to the gym, or going to the bathroom and seeing yourself in the mirror.

For Ada (introduced in Chapter 4), a long-term goal was to reduce the preoccupation with her skin. Ada had already picked going to work regularly as an exposure goal; therefore, she decided that her first response exercise would focus on the rituals related to going to work.

As you can see on the next page, Ada wrote down her rituals in much detail, which helped her set specific goals later on. Now it's your turn. Go ahead and fill in the columns in the worksheet.

Now that you've identified the rituals related to your long-term goal, you'll need to choose the specific ritual(s) you want to prevent. I suggest you start with just a few rituals (at the most three or four) that cause you no more than moderate distress (up to a rating of 60 at the most). You need to allow some flexibility and might need to work on fewer rituals if the rituals you're working with will be very hard to give up. The rule of thumb is that the more difficult it would be to prevent the ritual(s), the fewer rituals you want to choose for ritual prevention. To give you an idea of what we're trying to accomplish, take a look at what Ada did. She started by working on rituals related to her exposure and set a few short-term goals that were somewhat challenging but not overwhelming. Because she had so many rituals that related to her exposure—going to work—she needed to narrow her goals down further. So she decided that for 1 week she'd focus only on the rituals that occurred *before* work. It would have been too overwhelming to reduce simultaneously the rituals that occurred before and those that occurred at work.

Choosing a Ritual Prevention Strategy and Setting Short-Term Goals

After you choose the ritual you want to work on, you need to choose a ritual prevention strategy and set your ritual prevention goals. In a perfect world, you'd just rid yourself of all your rituals cold turkey. Once you're in the situation where the rituals would normally occur, you'd just stop them altogether. Obviously, this is the most efficient way of ridding yourself of unwanted rituals, and if it works for you, go ahead and do it! But don't be fooled; resisting rituals cold turkey is easier said than done. For many appearance rituals, it might not be possible. In these cases, you can use one of the more gradual approaches described below.

Selective Ritual Prevention: Picking Your Battles

Selective ritual prevention means you initially allow rituals only in certain situations and not in others. Again, you usually start with the rituals related to your most important major problem area. Most people who have avoidance behaviors

Trigger Situations Worksheet: Ada

Going to work	Distress if ritual was interrupted (0–100)	Frequency of rituals or time spent ritualizing
1. Before work: Washing face with soap and hot water	40	5 minutes
2. Before work: Inspecting appearance in the mirror, looking at face from different angles	60	40 minutes
3. Before work: Applying makeup	55	25 minutes
4. Before work: Asking husband for reassurance about appearance	50	4 times
5. At work: Comparing appearance to others' appearance	55	20 times
6. At work: Touching face to check for blemishes while sitting on desk	60	10 times
7. At work: Asking coworker Cara for reassurance	55	3 times
8. At work: Inspecting appearance in mirror	80	20 times
9. At work: Applying makeup	75	10 times

Trigger Situations Worksheet

	Distress if ritual was interrupted (0–100)	Frequency of rituals or time spent ritualizing

therefore begin by eliminating the rituals associated with the situations they've selected for exposures. If you have many rituals, you'll need to break down your short-term goals (that is, the rituals you want to prevent) even further. Ada reduced only the rituals before work as a first step. Other selective ritual prevention strategies you could consider might be to work on only certain rituals related to a particular exposure situation (for example, the least challenging ones) and leave the other rituals untouched for now.

Restricting Your Rituals: Watching the Clock

An excellent way to reduce ritualizing is to restrict the amount of time (or the number of repetitions) you allow for a particular ritual. If you choose this method, you first have to decide how much you want to reduce your ritual. Push yourself as much as you can, but also try to be realistic in judging what you can accomplish. For Ada this meant reducing the time for washing her face to 2.5 minutes (down from 5 minutes), as well as decreasing time for applying makeup to 4 minutes (down from 25 minutes). She chose these times because they were more in line with how long the average person would spend on those activities. She also decided to reduce the time for checking her appearance in the mirror to 15 minutes (from 40 minutes). Given that her distress rating for this situation was so severe and the urge to do the ritual was so strong, Ada felt this was the best she could do at the beginning.

She also decided to work on reassurance seeking, because her husband Jake was frustrated that she couldn't go to work without asking him several times, "How does my skin look?" Ada decided to cut this behavior down to once a day. Since this ritual also involved Jake, she told him of her new goal. Together, they decided that he'd answer her requests for reassurance only once before work. They also agreed that if she asked for reassurance more often, he'd respond (in a neutral voice): "Ada, we've agreed that I'll respond to this question only once before you go to work, and I've already done that for today." Telling others you trust about ritual prevention plans is a great strategy to help you stay on track. Chapter 11 provides some guidance for others who want to help you. Restricting the time (or the number of repetitions you allow for a ritual) is a very powerful ritual prevention strategy. You can just watch a clock or you may want to set a timer, and once the alarm goes off, whether you feel the ritual is complete or not, you'll have to stop.

Postponing a Ritual: When Procrastination Is a Good Thing

You can also get control over your appearance rituals by delaying them for a specific amount of time. You want to try to delay the ritual for as long as you possibly can. For some people this will be a minute, and for others, a day. So, for example, if you get the urge to go to the gym or to go to a tanning salon, plan on delaying this ritual for, say, 20 minutes. After 20 minutes, try to not give in to the ritual right away; rather, try to resist going again, this time perhaps for another 30 minutes, and then another 40 minutes, and so forth. How long you can postpone the ritual likely depends on the strength of the urge to do it.

If you have more than one ritual, start with the one that's easiest to delay. The delay will give you time to apply your cognitive strategies. For example, you could assess the pros and cons of ritualizing or evaluate the validity of the thoughts that caused the urge to ritualize. Using the cognitive strategies will often give you a different perspective, and you might find you no longer feel the need to ritualize when the time to ritualize arrives. Postponing is, of course, only an intermediate strategy to weaken the ritual; ultimately you'll have to stop the ritual altogether. In other words, even if you engage in skin picking or self-surgery a few hours later than you originally planned, you can still do a lot of damage. So eventually you should either delay the ritual to a point that's so far in the future that it does not happen at all or you have to combine this strategy with one of the other methods described here.

Making It Difficult for Your Ritual to Occur

Changing the Environment

An excellent strategy for reducing rituals involves making changes in your environment to decrease opportunities to carry out your ritual. This might mean avoiding some situations that can trigger your ritual (for example, don't go to a department store if one of your rituals is excessive spending on beauty products and clothing; stop touching your face if your ritual is picking at blemishes). It also means leaving a situation once a ritual starts (for example, Ada decided that she would leave the bathroom as soon as her allocated time for morning grooming was up). But you can stay in the situation if you change parts of the environment that make it hard to perform the ritual. For instance, some rituals require certain tools to carry them out. You might use a mirror to check your appearance, tweezers to pluck your facial hair or skin, or scissors to cut the hair on your head. Throwing out these tools, or making access to them more difficult, will automatically delay your ritual until you have access to the tools again. Gayle thought her lips were too thin. She didn't really have any avoidance behaviors, but she took her lipstick with her everywhere. When she started this program, she applied lipstick once or twice an hour. As a first step, she decided not to take the lipstick on shorter outings (for example, to the store). Aruna spent several hours a day tweezing little hairs from her face. She eventually told her mother to hold on to the tweezers and give them to her only every other day. Antonio was worried about hair loss and often attempted to count individual hairs. To control the counting, he put a lot of gel in his hair, which resulted in the hairs sticking together, thus making it impossible to count individual hairs. All of these strategies are called *stimulus control* by therapists, because you're controlling the triggering situation and surroundings.

Using Competing Actions

Any behavior that competes with the action of the ritual by using the same muscle groups for something else will make it difficult to perform a ritual. If you excessively pick at your skin to remove pimples, try making a fist whenever you feel the urge to ritualize. If the urges to pick usually occur while reading, hold the book tightly with both hands. If you get urges to ritualize while sitting in a chair, hold on to the arms of the chair. You could even carry a Koosh ball and squeeze it whenever the urge to pick occurs. It's important to maintain these *competing responses* for about 2 minutes, during which time your urges will likely decrease. If they don't, at least you had a little bit of time to think about strategies other than your ritual to deal with your urges (for example, perhaps you could select a cognitive strategy to deal with any distorted or unhelpful thoughts that may have come up in this situation). If you still have the urge to ritualize after using the competing response, try to engage in the competing response again, for another 2 minutes (in this sense, the competing response strategy is similar to postponing the ritual).

Combining Ritual Prevention Strategies and Finding Strategies That Fit Your Lifestyle

Whereas some people might be able to beat their rituals with just one of the preceding strategies, others do better mixing and matching. Ada combined selective ritual prevention (she initially focused only on rituals that occurred before work), restricting rituals (she cut down the time allowed for several rituals, as well as the number of repetitions for reassurance seeking), and stimulus control (she left her trigger situation as soon as she had completed the tasks she performed there). This shows how you can move from one strategy to another. It's important to figure out which techniques work best for you based on your specific ritual, your daily structure, your lifestyle, and where you are in this program. Optimally, your approach to ritual prevention should be socially inconspicuous, since this increases the likelihood that you'll actually use your strategies. However, if you live alone or with understanding family members or friends, you could even leave cues around the house that remind and motivate you to practice your ritual prevention exercises. Paste a sticky note on the bathroom mirror or on your exercise equipment that says "STOP IT" if you're having a problem with excessive mirror checking or exercise. If you experiment with one strategy and it doesn't work, try combining it—or following it—with another. Another important point to remember is that the strategies you're choosing should not be harmful (for example, you don't want to have a beer every time you try to postpone skin picking!). Don't replace one destructive behavior with another.

Increase Healthy Behaviors as You Decrease Your Rituals

Competing responses are just one example of how you can substitute unhealthy appearance rituals with more adaptive behaviors. Regardless of which ritual prevention strategies you choose, you should think of ways of increasing healthier activities. This is particularly important if you spent a lot of time ritualizing prior to starting this program. If you just cut down the rituals and do not fill the empty space they leave in your life, your rituals will creep back in before you know it. So think about activities that distract or prevent you from doing your rituals, and that may give you a sense of pleasure or mastery. Consider doing crossword puzzles, calling a friend, playing an instrument, doing woodwork, or cleaning the house. To increase healthy behavior, Ada decided to spend more time talking to her husband at the breakfast table before she left the house.

Go for It: Conducting Your First Response Prevention Exercise

Once you've selected your target rituals and given some thought to your ritual prevention strategy, you are almost ready to start completing your Exposure and Ritual Prevention (ERP) Worksheet. First, however, take a look at how Ada completed hers on the following page. In the first row, you can see that she was working on both exposure (going to work even if she thought she had some appearance flaws) and response prevention (decreasing appearance-related rituals before leaving the house). She also made sure she was aware of all rituals and avoidance behaviors associated with the situation on which she wanted to work. And she recorded her negative thoughts on a separate Thought Record and came up with more positive alternatives, which she included on her Exposure and Ritual Prevention Worksheet.

Ada was pretty distressed when she tried to get through the morning with only a few of her rituals, but she reached her goals, which gave her a little extra time to have a cup of coffee with her husband before leaving the house. This actually made her feel good about her practice. When she got to work, the most difficult moment was when she first saw her coworkers (as you can see, her distress rating actually goes up in the middle of the exposure), but after some time, she noticed that her feared consequences were not about to come true: Nobody stared at her. So she calmed down over the course of the day, and by the time she was ready to go home, she did not really feel distressed at all. Ada had reached

Exposure and Ritual Prevention Worksheet: Ada

My exposure and/or ritual prevention situation (be specific):
Decrease the rituals before going to work and don't avoid work even if I think that there's a problem with my looks.

What kind of avoidance behaviors or rituals do I need to watch out for?
Washing, face checking, excessive makeup application, reassurance seeking. Wanting to make excuses so that I don't have to go to work.

Preparing my thoughts:

Negative thoughts/predictions	Alternative thoughts
They'll see my large pores and zits! If my makeup is not perfect, everyone will stare at me.	They're not interested in my pores or my makeup. They're interested in how good a job I do at work!!
If my appearance is not perfect, I am flawed.	I'm not my pores or my blemishes. There is so much more to me than how I look.

Goals for the exposure and ritual prevention—How will I know I did well? (objective criteria):

1. Reduce time for washing face to 2.5 minutes
2. Reduce time for inspecting appearance in the mirror to 15 minutes
3. Reduce time for applying makeup to 4 minutes and apply less makeup
4. Leave bathroom after applying makeup, to decrease opportunities for ritualizing
5. Ask Jake for reassurance only once before going to work and tell him how I want him to respond to me
6. Increase time with Jake at the breakfast table instead; talk about fun stuff.

(continued)

136

Exposure and Ritual Prevention Worksheet: Ada *(continued)*

Distress rating:
Beginning: *60*
Middle: *65*
End: *5*

Evaluating my efforts:
Did I reach my goals?
Yes, all of them.

Did my negative thoughts/predictions come true?
No, nobody seemed to care.

What did I learn?
Maybe all of this avoidance and preparing is not necessary. People seem to respect me even if my pores and blemishes show a little. So maybe my pores and blemishes are not that important after all. If others can accept me like this, maybe I can, too.

How will I reward myself?
My husband actually rewarded me for trying to improve. He was very proud of what I had accomplished during my first ERP and gave me a massage. He's really glad that I am working on this, which makes me happy.

all of her goals for this day, and none of her negative predictions had come true, which led her to conclude that perhaps her blemishes and pores were not that important after all. She was also beginning to wonder whether more self-accep-tance was in order. Ada had involved her husband in the treatment, and he gave her a massage as a reward for working so hard in this program. Overall Ada's first ERP was a success.

Now it's your turn. Go ahead and complete your Exposure and Ritual Preven-tion Worksheet. As described, you want to start with situations that cause you moderate distress. Note all the avoidance behaviors and rituals associated with this situation, so you know what items need your attention. Next, try to anticipate your negative thoughts and develop alternatives (it will likely help you to use the Thought Record from Chapter 4 to develop some alternative thoughts). Then fill in your goals. As we discussed in Chapter 6, set goals that are *specific* and *objective* (goals focused on reducing time frames or number or repetitions meet all these cri-teria, because it's very easy to measure whether you achieve them), as well as *realis-tic* (push yourself, but don't set your expectations too high, or you might only end up frustrated). If you find that moderately distressing rituals are too difficult to work on right now, that's OK. Start with more manageable ones. Rate your distress right before you do ERP, then start your exercise.

After the ERP, rate your distress during and after the exercise. Review whether you reached your goals and record this in the appropriate space on the worksheet. Also remember to review the negative thoughts you had or predic-tions you made regarding the outcome of facing certain situations without ritu-als. Did the thoughts come true? Write down what you learned from the ritual prevention practice. Last but not least, don't forget to reward yourself!

Managing Your Anxiety during Response Prevention

When you first try a response prevention exercise, your distress rating might start out with a 50, and then it might drop. However, it could even go up to an 80 or a 90 as you continue to resist and have negative thoughts, then it will eventually drop down to a 70 or 60, until it finally ends up at 20, 10, or even 0. It's important not to give in to the ritual when your discomfort increases, because you then rob yourself of the opportunity to experience the decrease in distress you'll feel only if you work on the exercises long term. You might need all your willpower to do so. For the most part, people get out of this treatment whatever they put in to it. So if you're willing to tolerate some discomfort, the distress is pretty likely to go down. As we did with exposures, we approach response prevention gradually so you don't feel overwhelmed. Moreover, the cognitive strategies can prepare you for the ERP exercises and help you under-stand that many of your fears are not rational, and that your worst predictions usually don't come true.

Exposure and Ritual Prevention Worksheet

My exposure and/or ritual prevention situation (be specific):

What kind of avoidance behaviors or rituals do I need to watch out for?

Preparing my thoughts:

Negative thoughts/predictions   Alternative thoughts

Goals for the exposure and ritual prevention—How will I know I did well? (objective criteria):

1.

2.

3.

(continued)

Exposure and Ritual Prevention Worksheet *(continued)*

Distress rating:
Beginning:
Middle:
End:

Evaluating my efforts:
Did I reach my goals?

Did my negative thoughts/predictions come true?

What did I learn?

How will I reward myself?

How Much Time Should You Invest in Your Program?

In Chapter 6, I recommended that you invest at least 45–60 minutes per day in your program, and you should certainly continue to do so. Carry on with working on Thought Records and Exposures, and incorporate response prevention into the exercises you've conducted over the past few days.

In addition to working on those exercises you plan ahead of time, you'll now need to learn to respond flexibly to urges to ritualize whenever they occur. Urges to ritualize might be triggered at various times of the day and sometimes in situations where you did not expect them at all. So, at this point, in addition to conducting planned ERP, you'll need to learn to control your symptoms at all times of the day, basically whenever you feel the urge to ritualize. (Similarly, from this point forward you should also make a commitment to yourself that you will never again avoid a situation for which you have already conducted successful exposures.)

Practicing Ritual Prevention over the Course of Days and Weeks

Self-Monitoring

So far you've learned how to decrease a ritual in the context of a specific situation. Those situations usually will be exposures that you plan ahead of time. But for most people, rituals occur many times every day or every week. Therefore, as you move forward with your program, you'll also set goals that specify how often or how many times you allow a certain ritual on a given day, or in a given week. Indeed, your goals will often look like this: "Go to the gym only 3 times a week for 30 minutes each" or "apply lip balm only every 3 hours." While you should still complete an Exposure and Response Prevention Worksheet to help you work on those goals, you should also keep track of the frequency and duration of the targeted rituals on a self-monitoring sheet.

To get an idea of what self-monitoring looks like, take a look at Benito's example. Benito, a 41-year-old interior designer, thought his nose was "too fat." It was very difficult for him to meet with friends and clients, and he often canceled his appointments at the last minute. He had been working on not avoiding appointments for the last 3 days. His ritual prevention goal was to reduce mirror checking (or appearance checking in any other reflective surfaces) to less than 5 minutes per checking episode. He had originally also planned to completely stop comparing. Below you can see how he tracked various rituals related to his nose right before meeting with his friend Abel. As soon as he started self-monitoring, he quickly realized he was far from meeting his goals. Through self-monitoring he also became aware of thoughts and behaviors that he really had not noticed before, such as leaving a situation to check the mirror. So self-monitoring is not

Self-Monitoring Form for Appearance Rituals: Benito

Date/ Time	Trigger situation	Ritual	Thoughts	Feelings	Time spent ritualizing
8:20 am	Seeing myself in store windows when walking to my meeting with Abel	Inspecting nose from different angles	My nose is hideous! I'm so ugly!	Anxious, sad	On and off for 25 minutes
9:05 am	Looking at Abel's nose	Comparing myself	He's got such a strong and manly nose, and mine looks like a potato. He probably thinks I look like a clown. Why can't I look like him?	Ashamed	Over and over again for 30 minutes
9:25 am	Abel looked at me funny	Getting up and going to the bathroom mirror. Inspecting nose from different angles	He must have been really disgusted with my nose.	Anxious	5 minutes

only a good strategy to keep track of your rituals over time but it might also help you become aware of triggers, thoughts, and nuances of rituals. Benito addressed the thoughts he identified with Thought Records and revised his goals. Whereas some of his new goals were easier, he also decided that he'd never leave a social situation just to check a mirror. Thus, the more you know about your rituals, the better you can tailor your ERP strategy to your individual needs.

If your goals focus on reducing rituals that occur several times a day or week, you need to self-monitor to keep track of your progress. On your own self-monitoring form, please fill in the time your appearance rituals started, what triggered them, what the rituals were, the thoughts running through your mind, and the amount of time you spent ritualizing. Try to carry your monitoring logs with you wherever you go and, if possible, write the rituals down right after they occur (if that's not possible, write them down as soon as you get a chance). Besides learning more about your rituals, which will help you set better goals and keep track of your progress, there is an additional advantage to monitoring: For many people, monitoring itself is therapeutic and often decreases the frequency of rituals.

Structuring Your Program over Time

As discussed earlier, your program will likely start with an exposure that focuses on avoidance behavior related to the major problem area that causes you the most distress. Your first exposure situation should cause you only moderate distress. If you're performing many beauty rituals as well, exposure practice alone is not enough, and you'll need to incorporate response prevention into your exercises. It's also possible that you have only rituals, in which case your program will focus mainly on ritual prevention. Most people, though, have to practice both exposure and ritual prevention, which is why therapists commonly refer to ERP when talking about the techniques used in programs like this one.

To be sure that you've succeeded in a specific ERP situation, you should repeat it a few times, until your distress rating is reliably around 25 or lower. Initially you'll work on only one situation, but as soon as you've become a little more comfortable you should add more situations. Over the course of the next few weeks, you'll work your way up your distressing situations (to design exposures), as well as trigger situations, hierarchy (to design ritual prevention) step-by-step, so that your most challenging situations are completed in the latter part of the program. You want to be sure that you work on planned ERPs and Thought Records for at least 45–60 minutes per day. As I have already mentioned, it's really important that once you reach a certain goal, you maintain this standard (for example, once you've eaten in a brightly lit restaurant in a planned exposure, you cannot avoid it thereafter; once you've succeeded at leaving the house without sunglasses, you should not allow yourself to go back to wearing them). Thus, as you add more goals, you will ultimately make decreasing rituals

Self-Monitoring Form for Appearance Rituals

Date/ Time	Trigger situation	Ritual	Thoughts	Feelings	Time spent ritualizing

and facing your fears part of your daily life. Proceed with the program until you have mastered even the most difficult situations and rituals on your list.

To get an idea of how to change your ERP practice over the course of the program, take a look at Ada's ERPs completed at various stages. (Her first week of ERP corresponds to the fourth week of the overall BDD program, because she had to work on learning about BDD, assessments, and negative thoughts first.)

ERPs Ada Conducted during the First Week of ERP Practice

- Go to work regularly.
- Reduce time for washing my face to 2.5 minutes in the morning.
- Reduce time for inspecting my appearance in the mirror before work to 15 minutes.
- Reduce time for applying my makeup to 4 minutes in the morning and apply less makeup.
- Leave bathroom right after I apply makeup.
- Ask Jake for reassurance only once before going to work and tell him how I want him to respond to me.
- Increase time with Jake at the breakfast table instead; talk about fun stuff.

ERPs Ada Conducted during the Second Week of ERP Practice

- Reduce time for washing my face to 2 minutes in the morning.
- Reduce time for inspecting my appearance in the mirror before work to 4 minutes.
- Wear only mascara and lipstick (no facial makeup or concealer).
- Leave bathroom right after applying makeup.
- Don't ask Jake for reassurance.
- Increase time with Jake at the breakfast table instead; talk about fun stuff.
- No more comparing at work. Make sure to notice other non-appearance-related things about my coworkers.
- Don't touch my face to check while sitting at my desk.
- Go to church, sit in the front row.
- Meet friends for coffee or lunch at least every other day.

ERPs Ada Conducted during the Fourth Week of ERP Practice

- Reduce time for washing my face to 1 minute in the morning and 1 minute in the evening.
- Reduce time for inspecting my appearance in the mirror before work to 20 seconds.

- Wear only mascara and lipstick (no facial makeup or concealer).
- Leave bathroom right after applying my makeup.
- Don't ask anyone for reassurance.
- Spend more time with Jake and friends; talk about fun stuff.
- No more comparing at work or in any other social situations. Make sure to notice other non-appearance-related things about my coworkers.
- Don't touch my face at all.
- Decrease mirror checking to less than 10 minutes per day.
- Go to church, sit in the last row.
- Meet friends for coffee or lunch at least every other day.
- Wear shorts three times a week for at least 2 hours each.
- Shave only every other day for 5 minutes.

ERPs Ada Conducted during the Final Weeks of ERP Practice

- Reduce time for washing my face to 30 seconds in the morning and 30 seconds in the evening.
- Reduce time for inspecting my appearance in the mirror before work to 3 seconds.
- Wear only mascara and lipstick (no makeup or concealer); make sure to leave the house at least four times per week without any makeup at all.
- Don't ask anyone for reassurance.
- Spend more time with Jake and friends, talking about fun stuff. Meet friends for coffee or lunch at least every other day.
- Join a yoga class.
- No more comparing in any other social situations. Make sure to notice other non-appearance-related things about others.
- Don't touch my face.
- Do not check mirrors or take them anywhere; if I happen to see myself in a mirror somewhere, just look for 3 seconds at the most.
- Wear shorts three times a week for at least 2 hours each.
- Shave only every other day for 5 minutes.
- Go to church without any makeup; sit in the last row, shake hands with parishioners afterward, and look them right in the eyes.

Note how Ada worked on more and more challenging ERPs. She also worked on increasing healthier behaviors, such as spending more quality time with her husband and with friends, and starting a yoga class, and she continued working on her maladaptive thoughts on a daily basis. Note that by the fourth week of ERP, she had added the long-term goals that pertained to her second major problem area (the hair on her legs), and by the end of ERP she was working on all of her long-term goals listed in Chapter 4. Given that Ada approached her goals in such a structured manner, she was highly successful.

How Should You Evaluate Your Progress?

Just like Ada, you will be most successful if you approach your program in a systematic fashion. To stay on track, you'll need to evaluate your progress frequently. As described, you know you've successfully completed a particular ERP if you got your distress rating reliably around 25 or lower, you don't avoid the specific situation any longer, and you don't ritualize. So keep an eye on your self-monitoring logs and your ERP worksheets. Retake all the assessments from Chapter 4 about once a month and compare the goals you are currently working on with the long-term goals of the program. You know you're finished with the active phase of the program once you've reached all your long-term goals. When you've reached all those goals, you are ready for relapse prevention, described in Chapter 8.

Tailoring Your Program to Your Specific Rituals

An unlimited number of ritualistic behaviors occur in people with body image concerns, and most of them can be addressed in a straightforward manner with the strategies just described. However, there are also some rituals for which the strategies need to be adapted a little, specifically mirror checking, comparing, skin picking, excessive exercise, and cosmetic surgery.

Mirror Retraining: Seeing the Big Picture

Many people with appearance concerns dread looking in mirrors. They avoid mirrors because they're afraid of seeing their reflection. If you have a problem with mirrors, you may not look in mirrors at all, or you use only small or clouded mirrors. Or you avoid mirrors only when you're undressed. Or you might stare at your reflection for an hour or longer at a time. Some people alternate between checking mirrors over and over again and being unable to look in mirrors at all. Regardless of the nature of your problem with mirrors, you probably engage in some avoidance or ritualistic behavioral patterns that maintain your negative thoughts and feelings about your appearance. Read on, and you'll learn a new way of dealing with mirrors. The strategy described below was originally developed by Dr. James Rosen at the University of Vermont. I have modified it slightly and have since used it with hundreds of patients. This method is initially difficult, but be assured that it gets easier over time.

Ken, an attractive young real estate agent, enjoys his job and likes playing soccer. Nobody ever would guess that he hasn't been able to look in a clean, clear mirror for several months. When he brushes his teeth or combs his hair, he either walks away from the bathroom mirror or makes sure the light is dim and the mirror is foggy. When driving, he tries not to look in the rearview mirror. Ken is afraid to see his "long, bumpy nose." Many of his exercises in treatment have focused on working with mirrors.

Your work with mirrors will be similar to exposure practice, but it does much more than exposure: It retrains your perception. You need to remember a few important things when working with mirrors: First, try to find a mirror that's large enough to reflect your entire face (or if you have a problem with a body part other than your face, you need to use a full-length mirror). Keep the mirror in a well-lit area and try to stand as close to it as you can (about a foot away if you are working on your face, and about 3–4 feet away when working with a full-length mirror). When you first look in the mirror, you might have a tendency to focus mostly on the feature(s) you dislike. Over the course of this program, you will learn to broaden your perspective, so that you start paying attention to your other features as well. This will help to change how you perceive your appearance. Also, while looking in the mirror, you might get the urge to fix your appearance. Do not give in to this urge. The goal of this exercise is to learn to accept your appearance as it is, without changing it.

It took Ken several attempts before he could look in a clean mirror that was large enough to reflect his whole face. At first he was so uncomfortable that he could look in the mirror for only a couple of seconds. But he worked on it several times a day and gradually increased his time with every exercise he did. During the first few practices with the clean mirror, he focused only on his presumed defect. He conducted a 5-minute exercise but never paid attention to his nice blue eyes or his strong chin. He kept staring at his nose. But because he looked only at this one feature and not at others, his perception got distorted. This would happen to anyone who just kept staring at one thing for a very long time. After a while it just starts looking a little funny. That's why you have to remember not to spend any more time looking at your disliked features than at the rest of your face.

Ken not only had to work on looking at all of his facial features, but he also had to learn how to be more objective when thinking about them. For example, he had to stop calling his nose "grotesque." Instead he learned to describe it without judging it: "My nose is about 2½ inches long, and it has a slight elevation on the bridge."

You can learn to do the same. Look in the mirror and notice what you see. Again, don't prolong looking at the features that cause you problems, but don't avoid looking at them either. Also, don't stop the mirror exercise prematurely, even if you get uncomfortable. Just keep looking until the exercise is complete. As you're looking at your face, describe what you see. You can do this aloud or in your mind. Remember that it doesn't help you if you call a feature "hideous" or "ugly," or label yourself a "freak" or a "witch." If you catch yourself evaluating your appearance in such a negative way, stop, try to refocus on the exercise, and find a different, nonjudgmental descriptor. To ensure that you see your *entire* face, it may be helpful to look at your face (or body) systematically from top to bottom. As you see different features, try to describe them with *objective* terms. For example, you could start your objective body description with your hair. Describe its color and length. Move on to your forehead; describe the color of your skin and the shape, length, and color of your eyebrows. Next describe the color, shape, and size of your eyes and eyelashes, and do the same with your nose, ears, mouth, and chin. End with a detailed description of the shape of your face (or move on to the rest of your body).

So here is how Ken described his face after he had been working on it for a few days: "My hair is dark brown, and I have a crew cut. My forehead is a little tan, and I have two small wrinkles going horizontally across. They're both about a millimeter wide and couple of inches long. I also have a couple of vertical lines between the brows. My eyebrows are dark brown, almost black, and they are a little bushy, shaped a little like an arch, and about 2½ inches long. My eye color is blue, my eyelashes are black, and my eyes are almond shaped. They are about an inch and a half wide and almost an inch high. I have a couple of smile lines around both eyes. My nose is about 2½ inches long, and it has a slight elevation on the bridge. It's tan. My cheeks are tan and a little reddish on the cheekbones. I have three little acne scars on my left cheek and a couple of them on the right. They're small, maybe a couple of millimeters in diameter. My cheekbones are prominent. My ears are about 3 inches long and 2 inches wide. My lips are reddish, and my mouth is about 2 or 3 inches wide. My teeth are white; a couple of them are a little crooked. My chin protrudes a little, maybe a few millimeters. My face is oval."

The entire exercise should take about 5 minutes (if you describe your whole body it might take 10 minutes). Usually, at first it's quite anxiety provoking. Some patients even get a little nausea from being so uncomfortable. If this happens to you, just see it as a sign that you need to practice a little more. Be patient. It will get easier. It's also very easy to fall into your old habits and judge your appearance instead of just describing it. So watch out. You don't want to evaluate, just describe. If you had a problem standing close to your mirror at first, you can now work on that as well. Over the next few days, try to stand closer to the mirror. Let's say you started by keeping a distance of 3 feet between you and the mirror; try to reduce the distance to 2 feet the next day. Again, these exercises can be quite uncomfortable initially, but they'll get easier after you have repeated them a few times. A good variation of this exercise is to do it with someone you trust. This support person could even hold the mirror for you and move it closer to your face as you get more comfortable. In addition, he or she could stop or correct you if you're using judgmental terms to describe your looks.

Now let's examine how somebody who has problems with her thighs reduced her problems with mirror avoidance. Pam, a popular college student, is smart and has a great sense of humor. Although in reality she's not less attractive than other women, she often thinks she is. Pam is convinced that her thighs are "too white and too fat." Plus she has a little scar on her right knee from an accident, which she really dislikes. There are many things that she doesn't do because of her appearance concerns, such as wearing shorts, exercising, and shopping for clothes. She avoids the gym and the mall because there are "too many mirrors." Pam thinks she looks "OK" when she's wearing a long flowing skirt, but she can't bear to look in the mirror when she's wearing only underwear or is undressed.

Pam had to learn to look at herself from head to toe instead of just focusing on her legs. She also had to learn to be more objective and specific: "My thighs are 20 inches round" rather than "They're disgusting and fat." Or "I have a scar on my right knee; it's about 1 inch long and pink" instead of "I'm disfigured." Here are some of the mirror retraining exercises Pam worked on over the course of the program:

- Look at my entire body in the mirror, wearing just shorts and a tank top (since Pam had a problem with her thighs, she used a full-length mirror to complete her exercises).
- Look at my naked body in the mirror.
- Exercise on treadmill in the gym twice per week, wearing shorts; look in mirrors while I'm exercising.

Of course, she wanted her mirror retraining work to be maximally beneficial in terms of changing her distorted perception to a more accurate view of herself. Therefore, when doing these exercises, she tried to be objective, specific, and nonjudgmental when describing her body. Sometimes her goals were quite challenging, and if she felt overwhelmed, she'd break them down into smaller, more manageable ones. For example, the first time she worked on wearing only shorts in front of the mirror, she was really worried about seeing the scar and stood about 6 feet from the mirror. Over time she gradually came closer.

Changing a Narrow Focus: How to Battle Comparison Rituals

The large majority of people with body image problems have comparison rituals. Unfortunately, the more you compare yourself to others, the worse your appearance obsession gets. Stewart, a tall, dark, handsome pilot, strongly believes that looking good is an important part of being successful in today's world. That's why he exercises almost daily and spends quite a bit of money on brand-name clothing. But he thinks his cheekbones are too red and asymmetrical, and he constantly compares his cheekbones to those of other guys. When I asked him how time-consuming this was, he replied: "It's constant. Especially if I'm around people I haven't met before, like in a restaurant, it goes on nonstop. Depending on where I am, it could go on for up to 8 hours a day. I just keep comparing and comparing and comparing." This usually causes him to feel like a failure. He feels envious of others who looked better and is jealous whenever his girlfriend talks to a guy with cheeks he considers better than his own. While most of the time his comparisons are limited to cheekbones, occasionally he compares himself with respect to body build or other physical aspects. But even if he sees a guy who is a bit out of shape or overweight, he just takes this as a reminder of what would happen if he let himself go.

Stewart overcame his comparison ritual with a number of strategies. To expand his focus from the area of his body he hated so much to other things in life, he needed to learn to turn on all of his senses rather than just getting hung up on one thing. In a restaurant, this meant, for example, paying attention to the taste of the food, the conversation, the smells, or the sound of the music. When talking to others, he also learned to pay attention to characteristics besides appearance (for example, the sound of friends' voices, their sense of humor, interests, struggles). Broadening his focus ultimately helped him overcome his comparing ritual, and because he started to pay more attention to whatever his friends and coworkers were saying (rather than just focusing on their looks), it actually made him more popular as well. Others found him more fun, more entertaining, and more relaxed in social situations. At the end of this program, Stewart said that for the first time in years he actually felt like he was enjoying social situations again.

Dealing with Skin Picking

Ofir, a smart 24-year-old college student, is bright, gets good grades, has many friends, and is for the most part pretty social. Only his family members know how much he used to struggle with his skin. As soon as he saw a little imperfection, he felt compelled to pick at it. His skin was actually not bad, but he had a few bumps and blackheads. He picked at them for long periods of time and felt satisfied only when he "got something out." He usually started by standing in front of a bathroom mirror, touching his skin to figure out whether there were any bumps. As soon as he found some kind of imperfection, he'd turn up the light in the bathroom, sit on the sink to get a closer look, and start picking with his fingernails. Within minutes, he'd move on to using tweezers, or even needles or pins to clean out his skin. His picking was an attempt to improve his appearance, but after a skin-picking episode he usually felt terrible. He thought he had really "made a mess" and regretted that he had touched his skin in the first place. He then tried repairing his skin by applying lotions. Sometimes he felt so bad about having damaged his skin that he could leave the house only after applying concealer. At other times he felt so ashamed that he could not leave the house at all.

If you have a similar problem, you may pick at your skin until it's red and swollen. You may not stop at your face but may also pick at your back or arms. You may pick your skin before you leave the house, when you think there's a pimple, or every night before you go to bed. Skin-picking rituals are different from normal grooming, because they are very time-consuming and cause tissue damage. A similar issue is tweezing or pulling your hair. You may look for facial or neck hair to pull out, over and over again, hundreds of times a day, and still not feel that you're done. Excessive skin picking and hair tweezing (or hair cutting) generally responds well to stimulus control, restricting your rituals, competing responses, and postponing. Let's take a look at what Ofir did to get his skin-picking problem under control.

One typical thought Ofir tended to have when he saw or felt an imperfection on his skin was that he needed to pick his skin to improve it. The alternative thought he prepared with the strategies from Chapter 5: "This is not true. Nothing bad is going to happen to me if I leave my skin alone. But if I do pick at it, I'll do some damage and feel guilty and ashamed afterward." A typical thought Ofir tended to have after a picking episode was "If I go out after picking, everyone will see what I've done!" And the alternative thought he prepared was "So what! Other people don't have perfect skin either, and they still go out and have fun!" When Ofir first came to me, he picked about two or three times on an average day—in the morning before leaving the house, sometimes at school in the bathroom, and at night before going to bed. The morning skin-picking episodes lasted about 10–15 minutes; the school episodes lasted 5 minutes, and the episodes at night lasted 25–40 minutes. On weekends, however, before he went out to meet his friends, Ofir's picking could easily take an hour and was quite distressing. Although Ofir really hated the picking episodes on the weekends most, he decided it was too hard to reduce them as a first treatment target. He was pretty confident, however, that he could cut down the rituals that occurred on workdays. So in one of his early ERPs Ofir decided to (1) decrease the morning picking episodes to 7 minutes, (2) stop picking completely at school, (3) reduce night picking to 15 minutes, and (4) completely rid himself of avoidance behavior (for example, not leaving the house after a bad episode) that occurred during the course of the week.

Ofir was very successful with working on his rituals. His original plan was to restrict his morning ritual to 7 minutes, but he ended up using a competing response—he made a fist—and kept postponing the picking in 5-minute increments. Eventually he went to school without having picked at all! He was successful at stopping the school-picking ritual cold turkey. The nighttime ritual was the most difficult one to control. He had been trying to avoid the bathroom, where he usually picked as much as possible. Just in case, he had also put sticky notes on the bathroom mirror, which read: " Picking is going to make it worse!" and "Stop! I can resist." He tried not to turn up the light in the bathroom and avoided sitting on the sink. He had even thrown out his tweezers. All these strategies helped him stay away from the mirror for some time. Eventually he got sucked toward the mirror anyway, but after 12 minutes, he started to use his competing response (he moved his hands away from his face and made a fist), and he also reminded himself of his alternative thoughts. This helped him stop the ritual right away. As he had planned, he also conducted an exposure and went for a walk right after he picked.

Ofir's story provides you with a nice example of how combining several ritual prevention strategies can lead to success, and Ofir ultimately felt very good about his exercise. To reward himself for his good work, he had dinner at his favorite Mexican restaurant. Over the course of the following week, he further reduced the morning and nighttime rituals. Finally, as a last step in his program, he also mastered his weekend rituals. Ofir completed his program over 3 years ago, and although he still occasionally picks at his skin, he feels much more in control and is very satisfied with his progress.

Muscle Dysmorphia: Excessive Exercise and Steroids

Owen is an accountant in his early 30s. He is tall and handsome, and is one of the biggest guys I know. Nevertheless, he feels like he is "too small" and does "not look manly enough." "I am obsessed with the gym," he confessed, "especially lifting. It's hard for me to think about anything else. I've got in trouble many times at work because I got stuck in the gym during lunch break and was late for meetings by the time I got back. I miss out on so many things others look forward to, like spending time with my girlfriend, family functions, or meeting friends, because I feel I need the time to work out. My girlfriend thinks I'm crazy because of the amount of time I spend at the gym and all the fuss I make about eating healthy. I haven't even told her about the other stuff, like the steroids." Indeed, much of Owen's income goes toward dietary supplements and even occasionally black-market anabolic steroids to make himself look more muscular.

In addition to being concerned about his overall body size, Owen felt that his penis was too small. He spent a lot of time reading about diets, exercise, and all sorts of ways to improve his looks. Because he was so self-conscious about his "small" appearance, he'd never take off his clothes in the locker room. On days when he felt particularly bad about his appearance, he wore multiple layers of clothing or even padded his clothes and underwear to make himself look bigger.

Owen suffered from a problem called *muscle dysmorphia*, which is basically the belief that one is too small and not muscular enough. Fortunately, he recognized that something was really wrong and decided to start a CBT program much like the one described in this book. Early on, it became obvious that Owen kept comparing himself with steroid-pumping Hollywood hunks who had bodies much larger than Mother Nature had ever intended them to be. Thus, he always felt like he didn't measure up. After addressing some of his negative thoughts about his appearance with the strategies outlined in Chapter 5, his first treatment goal was to eliminate completely the anabolic steroid use. He chose this as his first treatment target, because anabolic steroids can have pretty serious side effects, such as acne, sleep disturbance, high blood pressure and high cholesterol, impotence, depression, increased aggression, impassivity, and liver disease. Moreover, if used long-term, steroids become addictive. Since Owen hadn't used steroids regularly, it was relatively easy to stop them. Unlike many other users who decide to quit, he did not experience withdrawal symptoms.

As the next treatment goal, Owen restricted his exercise routine to 1.5 hours per day. Since he now had some additional free time, he began to coach a soccer team for young boys. This allowed him to stay involved with sports and physical fitness, but from a much more fun perspective. Over the next few weeks he was able to decrease his rituals further, until he eventually worked out only three to four times a week for about 40 minutes each time.

In the second week of his program, Owen started reviewing his dietary supplements and the amount of money he spent on them. Because he had lost track of what's normal and what others do with respect to eating, he asked three of his friends (who did not have a problem with their body image) about their eating habits and their use of supplements. It surprised him how little they cared about vitamins, protein intake, and so forth. So he decided to cut down the supplements gradually by eliminating one a day. Using the strategy of stimulus control, he also canceled his subscriptions to bodybuilder magazines, which dramatically reduced the time he spent reading about exercise. As he decreased his ritualistic behaviors, he also increased exposure to situations he had been avoiding. For example, for exposure practices, he set goals such as wearing no padding and fewer and fewer layers of clothing to family functions or other social events. As he felt more comfortable with these exercises, he worked on changing clothes in a locker room and, finally, walking around on a beach in a bathing suit.

I hope Owen's story gives you some ideas for dealing with muscle dysmorphia. Keep in mind that a self-help treatment is not sufficient if you use steroids regularly, or if you have exercised to the point that you have already damaged your body. In this case you need to work with clinicians who are knowledgeable about muscle dysmorphia and steroid abuse. This is important to prevent (further) medical complications. The book *The Adonis Complex* by Drs. Harrison G. Pope, Jr., Katharine A. Phillips, and Roberto Olivardia might also be very useful if you suffer from muscle dysmorphia (see Resources).

Plastic Surgery and Dermatological Treatments

Lorenzo is a 36-year-old father of three and a successful business owner. In general he seems like a happy guy, so most of his customers would never know how much he suffers because of his looks. However, Lorenzo thinks that his nose is too bumpy, his skin is too pimply, and his hair is too thin. He always envies other guys who have strong, straight noses, better skin, or more hair. He has been in dermatological treatment for supposedly bad skin since his teens and has been using hair growth tonics since he was 25.

At 26, Lorenzo had his first nose job. His wife told me: "I was really against the surgery at first. . . . It seemed so much more radical than the kind of stuff he usually did to deal with his appearance obsessions. . . . But he was so unhappy, so eventually I told him to just go ahead. What a terrible mistake! Although I liked his new nose after the surgery, Lorenzo was convinced that the surgeon had really screwed up. That he took too much off or something. . . . So after the surgery, Lorenzo felt even worse about his nose than he did before. He was getting really depressed and didn't want to leave the house. The worst part was that he kept blaming himself for having gone forward with the surgery. At some point he even had an idea to sue the surgeon, but I was able to stop him from that. So we went ahead and scheduled a second surgery with another surgeon, who had a really good reputation. Again, things were worse rather than better after the operation. Then Lorenzo had a third nose job and was again devastated by the results. At that point, I was getting really fed up with all this. I finally put my foot down and told him I'd leave him if he didn't stop with all those surgeries. I also insisted that he get psychiatric treatment. So he started cognitive-behavioral therapy. That's when things started to improve. . . ."

Lorenzo's story is not unusual. Many people with body image problems seek repeated medical remedies or procedures to deal with their supposed defects. The list of procedures is endless and includes visits to dermatologists for acne, scarring or presumed redness or paleness of the skin, laser hair removal or visits to endocrinologists for too much (or too little) body hair, visits to dentists for braces, to urologists for penis enlargement, to plastic surgeons for nose jobs or breast enlargement, and so forth.

Cosmetic surgery is increasingly common and one of the most extreme procedures to deal with body image concerns. Whereas many people are very satisfied with the outcome of cosmetic surgery, others are extremely disappointed. So keep in mind that surgery is not for everyone, and the reason you might want surgery is one of the most important predictors of your satisfaction. Therefore, if you are planning on scheduling surgery, evaluate your expectations and your motivation very carefully. The more radical the procedure you are considering, the more carefully you need to weigh the pros and cons of this step.

Based on my clinical experience and preliminary research in this area, I usually discourage people who suffer from BDD from undergoing surgery. This is because the large majority of my BDD patients were dissatisfied with the results of their surgery, despite the fact that the outcome was objectively fine. Keep in mind that surgery can change only your appearance, not what's inside. If you have BDD, you need psychiatric treatment, not a face-lift. But even if you don't meet the full criteria for BDD, if you have unrealistically high expectations, you're setting yourself up for a big disappointment. Pay close attention when reading or talking to others about limitations of surgery. Most likely, surgery is not going to turn you into a supermodel, and there might be less improvement with surgery than you initially expected. If you tend to change your appearance frequently, you may want to hold off on an irreversible procedure like surgery. Certainly you never want to pursue cosmetic surgery to please someone else. You are the only person who can decide whether you need surgery. Also, if you assume that surgery is going to change your life in a major way (that you'll be a lot more popular or find a new lover; that you'll get married; or that your unfaithful spouse will return to you), you are most likely headed for disappointment.

Your expectations should also be realistic in terms of time away from work and social activities, physical discomfort or pain, financial cost, and medical risks and complications. Don't just think "I'll have it done now, and I'll worry about how to pay for it later!" or "I won't have these medical complications." Cosmetic surgery is real surgery, so there are substantial costs. And there are risks such as infection, bruising, swelling, skin death, or asymmetry after surgery. All of these factors can impact your satisfaction with the surgery outcome. Sensory changes (for example, numbness, tingling) at the surgery site can occur as well. If you are not willing to consider the disadvantages of surgery, you may be headed for a rude awakening.

If you have indeed considered all the pros and cons and are still on the fence about surgery, let me make a suggestion. Hold off with surgery and other medical treatments related to your body image concerns and give this program a good try for 12 weeks or so (it may take longer if your body image problems are more severe). Work on your appearance-related thoughts, beauty rituals, and avoidance behaviors. If you are like most of the patients I've worked with, you won't feel the need for cosmetic surgery or similar procedures at the end of the program.

What's Next?

If you have not done any ERPs by the time you read this, you really need to get going right now. Get yourself an Exposure and Ritual Prevention Worksheet, fill out the top section, and get to work on your first ERP! To be successful, you'll have to do many ERPs over the next few weeks.

Chapter 8

Getting at Your
Core Beliefs

During the first few weeks of this program, you've been working on changing relatively superficial thoughts triggered by specific situations, such as "The sales clerk in the store this afternoon kept looking at my scar," while also doing increasingly challenging behavioral exercises. By now, however, you've likely noticed that certain beliefs or themes occur over and over on your Thought Records. Some of those thoughts might take the form of rigidly held assumptions, such as "My appearance is more important than my personality, my skills, and my intelligence." Dr. Judith Beck calls those rules or assumptions intermediate-level beliefs. Intermediate beliefs might be expressed as if–then statements, such as "If my appearance is defective, then I am worthless" or "If I don't find a way to improve my appearance, then I'll never get married." They might also take the form of "should" statements—"I should look perfect at all times"—because often the implicit assumption is "If I don't look perfect, I'm inadequate."

Dr. Beck calls the deepest levels of beliefs *core beliefs*. They are overgeneralized global beliefs about yourself, your future, or the world around you, like "I'm defective," "I'm bad," "I'm worthless," "I'm unlovable," "I'm a loser," "The odds are against me," and "You can't trust anyone." These deeper-level beliefs are usually learned in childhood and are still active later in life, whether there's any supporting evidence for them or not. As mentioned in Chapter 5, core beliefs might be a result of what you picked up from the people around you (for example, if your parents based their own self-worth on appearance, you might have learned to do the same). Negative, self-defeating core beliefs can also develop after certain experiences that affect your self-esteem, such as abuse, discrimination, or teasing.

Core beliefs are unconditional. They filter your perception and therefore affect how see yourself or others in specific situations. So, for example, if you think you're defective, you'll judge everything that's happening to you based on this belief. You might assume that people in specific situations react negatively to you, and you'll avoid certain social situations. *Changing at a deeper level will address the root culprit of your negative thinking.* This will have a positive effect on the way you feel about yourself and will help you let go of self-defeating behaviors. It will also help you maintain the improvements you make with this program. In this chapter, I show you how to modify those outdated deeper-level beliefs and develop healthier ones to replace them. I'll also show you how to widen the lens through which you view yourself and the world. Instead of basing your self-worth on a few appearance-related details, you'll learn to see yourself in a much broader context, one that expands your horizons and your ability to enjoy life.

When to Start Working on Deeper-Level Beliefs

The time to start working on deeper-level beliefs is after you've completed many Thought Records, done your first few ERP exercises, and made some progress in mirror retraining. This usually occurs around week 5–6, once you've successfully modified negative thoughts triggered by specific situations that occur in your day-to-day life. But even if by week 7 you still have trouble believing the rational responses that you write down on your Thought Records, you should start addressing core beliefs, too. In this chapter, you'll learn how to identify and modify those deeper-level beliefs.

Identifying Assumptions and Core Beliefs

A good way to identify deeper-level beliefs is to review your Thought Records and ERP worksheets. Ask yourself if there are any themes on those records that occur over and over again. For example, when Peter reviewed his Thought Records, he kept finding beliefs such as "I'm not handsome enough" or "I can't do anything right." These thoughts pretty clearly seemed related to the deeper-level belief "I'm inadequate."

Another way to identify deeper-level beliefs is the *downward arrow technique*. This widely used technique has been described by many authors, including Drs. Christine A. Padesky and Dennis Greenberger, as well as by Dr. David D. Burns. To use this method, just select one of your thoughts on a Thought Record that you suspect may be related to a deeper-level belief. Then repeatedly ask the following questions, "What does this say about me?" or "And if this were true, what would be so bad about it?"

Nadda is excessively concerned that her eyebrows are not plucked perfectly. She checks the mirror for a total of 2 or 3 hours a day and won't leave the house if she thinks her eyebrows are imperfect. Take a look at how Nadda applied the downward arrow technique.

I think I plucked too many eyebrows last time, and now they are too thin.
(What's so bad about that?)
↓
If anyone notices, they will think how bad I look.
(What's so bad about that?)
↓
If they think I look bad, they will reject me.
(What so bad about that?)
↓
I will never find anyone who will love me.
(What does this say about me?)
↓
I'm unlovable.

Nadda stopped the downward arrow once she reached a belief that seemed absolute. Most of the time, my patients use this strategy to identify beliefs about themselves (usually starting with "I am . . ."). However, you can also use this strategy to identify beliefs about others ("What does this say about Joe?") or the world around you ("What does this say about how the world operates?").

Once you've identified a deeper-level belief, you can use the following strategies to weaken old, unhelpful beliefs. While you modify old self-defeating beliefs, you can also strengthen healthier new assumptions and core beliefs.

Changing Assumptions Related to a Narrow Appearance Focus

Broadening your perspective from your perceived appearance flaw to other characteristics of yourself (and even other aspects of life) is one of the main goals of this program. You already did some work on this when you learned to pay attention to your body as a whole during the mirror retraining exercises in Chapter 7. You also learned to look at others more holistically when you worked on comparing rituals, also in Chapter 7. Your exposure exercises from Chapter 6 should have shown you that even if you participate in life more fully without hiding your flaws, others are still just as caring and accepting. These experiences can have a powerful effect on your evaluation of the importance of your looks. Most people also change their views pertaining to the importance of appearance as a natural consequence of applying the thought management strategies in Chapter 5. They learn to put things in perspective and ask themselves questions like "Is it really true that this situation has anything to do with my skin?"; "What is actually important about this situation?"; and "In the meeting with my boss, is it more important that I can present the sales figures from the last quarter or that my pores look small?" So, over the course of this program, you have already taken several steps to broaden your perspective from your preoccupation with your perceived flaw to a more balanced view of life. In the next step, you'll learn how you can change the deeper-level beliefs related to your narrow focus on appearance.

Writing a Letter to Your (Imagined) Children

Many of my patients have rules for themselves that they'd never impose on anyone else. Nadda held the belief, "I should leave the house only when my eyebrows are plucked perfectly and my makeup is just right. If my appearance is flawed, others won't like me." Nadda's rules and assumptions about others resulted in the many hours she spent in front of the mirror. They also led her to avoid situations on days that she didn't meet her high appearance standards. In treatment, I encouraged Nadda to pretend she had a daughter who spent many hours a day fixing her eyebrows and makeup because she was afraid others would reject her if her appearance were not perfect. I encouraged Nadda to write a letter providing advice and guidance to her imagined child. Here's what she wrote:

Dear Daughter:

I know how afraid you are to face the world. But it's not a good idea to spend so much time on fixing and hiding your appearance. These rituals will only keep alive your belief that your appearance dictates whether others like you. You need to put this belief to the test. Stop the camouflaging and see what happens. I doubt anyone will reject you, because they don't care about your makeup and eyebrows as much as you do. But you'll have to face this fear for yourself, so you can learn it's unjustified. Show the world who you really are. You have so many talents and qualities you can be proud of and others can love you for. You are a warm and loving person, a great listener, a wonderful artist, and such a good cook! If you stop hiding and face the world without being so made up, you'll see that it's really you they care about.

Love,
Mom

Nadda found that writing this letter helped her develop more rational assumptions about what people care about in others—assumptions that she could then apply to herself. Many people also find that their rules change when they are imposing them on others. The benefit of this distance makes it easier for them to be more tolerant toward themselves. But if you don't think this would work for you, try the next strategy.

Considering What You Respect in Others

Rafael, a 38-year-old bank teller, has been very concerned about signs of aging, especially the wrinkles around his eyes. He's afraid others will see him as old and therefore respect him less. He worries about how the light hits his face in social situations and spends several hours a day checking the mirror. He also applies many creams and lotions to his skin. The belief that caused him the most agony was "If anyone sees my wrinkles, they'll think less of me!"

He considered his appearance more important than his intelligence, personality, or skills. On top of that, Rafael had very high standards for his looks and as a result frequently felt ashamed because he felt he couldn't live up to them. In treatment, he found it particularly helpful to shift his perspective by asking himself these questions:

> "If I noticed that one of my colleagues had wrinkles, what would I think of him? Would I respect him less? What are the characteristics I respect people for?"

> "Are there other people I respect who have wrinkles? How concerned are they about their wrinkles? Are they less ashamed? Why?"

Answering these questions helped him develop this rational response: "Ernesto, who is the person I like and respect the most in my company, has wrinkles, and he doesn't seem to care about them at all. I don't respect others for their appearance, but rather for their accomplishments, values, and skills. And I think others respect me for the same things: for my hard work, good leadership skills, and good social manners." Changing his perspective helped Rafael accept his wrinkles and realize they were not important. This shift in attitude also had a major impact on this mood: He felt less ashamed and more confident.

As I mentioned earlier, broadening your perspective from your appearance to other characteristics of yourself (and even other aspects of life) is one of the main goals of this program. So if you have an assumption similar to Rafael's, complete a Thought Record and ask yourself questions that focus on the importance of appearance in your evaluation of others. Think of your role models or people you consider leaders, or simply consider the people in your life that you respect the most. Is your respect based on their appearance, or are there other traits and accomplishments? If so, which ones? Do you have any of the traits you respect in others? If so, which ones? Just like Rafael, write them in the "Rational response" section of a Thought Record.

Starting at the End

A few years back, my patient Zabia told me she would not even consider reducing her hairstyling ritual to less than 1 hour a day. She said: "There's no way I could face my friends and coworkers with messy hair! It's really important to me that my hair look stylish! I just don't want them to think badly of me!" She was often late for work and family events because she had to fix her hair. And on days when she could not get it right, she did not want to leave the house at all. This led to many arguments with her husband, who would have liked to go out with her more often. With the downward arrow technique I described earlier, we quickly determined that Zabia's thoughts and behavior were driven by the assumption, "If my hair is not perfect, others won't like me!" So I asked Zabia, "Let's assume that you had a long successful life and you are now lying on your deathbed. As you are looking back at your life, what kind of memories do you want to have?" Zabia thought about her answer for a long time. Then she replied: "I want to think of the many beautiful moments I spent with friends and family. I want to remember fun, laughter, intimacy, and closeness. And I want to travel, you know, and not just in the United States. So I want to remember all the different and exotic places I have seen. I guess the most important thing would be that I would look back at a life that's filled with many meaningful experiences!" Next I asked Zabia, "Now, let's pretend that after your death, you're watching your own funeral. . . . What would you want people to say about you?" She told me the following: "I want people to say that I was a caring person. I want to be a mother one day, you know, and I want my children to say that I was a really great mom. I want my husband to say that I was a loving wife. And because I'm a teacher, I would want people to acknowledge that I made a contribution to the lives of the kids in my classes. I guess I'd like people to say that, in my own way, I made the world a little better." Zabia started laughing when I pointed out that she never mentioned that she wanted to have memories of hours and hours in front of the mirror trying to get her hair just right. Also, she did not even care to be remembered for her stylish hair!

Now it's your turn. Think about the end of your life and ask yourself what kind of memories you want to have? How do you want to be remembered? Write your answers down, because they will give you a more balanced view of how important your appearance really is compared to other things in life.

Your Self-Esteem Pie: Broadening Your Focus

Elena has had problems with low self-esteem as long as she can remember. Over the course of her program, she addressed thoughts that related to being too short and having a scar on her face. She also completed some ERPs on not wearing heels and leaving the house without makeup. Although she made progress, after 7 weeks Elena was still struggling quite a bit in certain social situations. Her downward arrow technique revealed the belief, "I am inadequate." To assess the impact that her body image had on her self-worth, she completed a self-esteem pie. She drew a circle and divided it up in different pieces. As you can see below, the pieces represent the components of her self-esteem, both positive and negative.

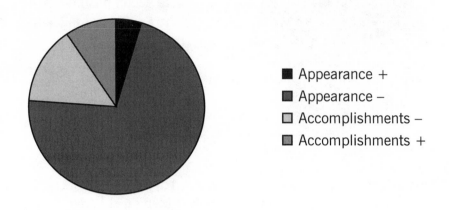

About 80% of Elena's self-esteem was based on her appearance. And what's worse, about 75% percent of these appearance evaluations were negative and only 5% were positive. Elena also based part of her self-worth on her accomplishments. She had more negative (15%) than positive (10%) feelings about those. Overall, her self-image was more negative than positive. Obviously, Elena was hard on herself when completing this chart. For example, her negative appearance evaluation was mostly due to her height and her scar. The only positive feature she had thought of were her breasts. She did not even consider her beautiful white teeth, her expressive eyes, her full lips, or her attractive figure. In the area of achievements, she put herself down because she had dropped out of graduate school—even though she had dropped out because her daughter had a serious illness and needed to be cared for at home. She didn't give herself much credit for being a good mom and having successfully raised two children. When completing this chart, she also didn't think much about the fact that she had started her own retail business from scratch 3 years earlier. Nor did she consider that she was actually pretty smart and had an outstanding memory. Finally, Elena did not factor personality or talent into her self-evaluation. She took it for granted that she had many friends and had a beautiful singing voice.

After Elena's therapist encouraged her to list some positive appearance features, her achievements, and her personality traits, she began seeing herself differently. She was able to recognize her skills, abilities, and successes. Based on these new insights, Elena decided to revise her self-image pie a little. First she decreased the negative appearance slice; this made room for larger positive achievement, intelligence, personality, and accomplishment slices. Her new self-esteem pie looks like this:

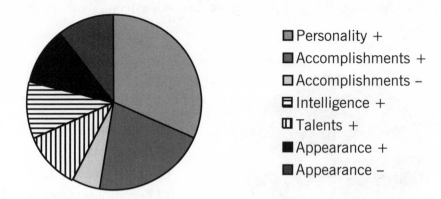

Personality +
Accomplishments +
Accomplishments –
Intelligence +
Talents +
Appearance +
Appearance –

Decreasing the importance of her perceived appearance defects and recognizing her many other positive qualities helped Elena feel better about herself. To ensure that she would remember this exercise, she not only kept her new self-esteem pie on the refrigerator but she also wrote down all her positive qualities under "evidence that contradicts old core belief, 'I'm inadequate'" on her core belief record and came up with the new core belief, "I'm OK."

Questions to Help You Develop More Positive Self-Esteem

Like Elena, most of us have strengths in some domains, shortcomings in others, and are average in most areas. If you overfocus on your limitations (while perhaps at the same time not recognizing your assets), your self-esteem will be low. Therefore, it's important that you put your imperfections in perspective and evaluate yourself more holistically. Don't base your entire self-worth on one domain, such as appearance. If you do this, even a tiny scar or pimple can send you into a crisis. To help you broaden your perspective, I'd like to encourage you to think of as many potential assets in different areas as you can. Take a look at the following list of questions to help you find those assets:

- **Intelligence:** Do you generally comprehend things? Are you able to solve problems? Do you know trivia? Do you have a good vocabulary? Have you ever explained things to others or helped them with something? Can you focus on the task at hand? Do you have a good memory?
- **Accomplishments/competence:** What do/did you do well? Is there anything you are proud of? Have others ever complimented you for something? Have you ever been promoted or honored in any way? Do you have

skills around the house, such as cooking, gardening, entertaining, decorating, and so forth?

- **Creative and artistic abilities:** Do you write poetry, sing, play an instrument, paint, and so forth?
- **Athletic abilities and health:** Do you exercise or play a sport? Are you fit, strong? Are you physically healthy?
- **Work habits:** Do you work hard? Are you prepared? Do you arrive on time, meet deadlines, take short breaks, and so forth?
- **Relationships:** Do you have any strength that others would appreciate in a relationship? Do you have any good relationships (for example, friends, parents, children, siblings, colleagues, classmates)? In challenging relationships, are there aspects that are positive? What do you contribute to those positive aspects?
- **Personality:** What qualities do others like or respect about you? Are you friendly, kind, loyal, compassionate, caring, generous, polite, respectful, reliable, responsible, persistent, and witty? Do you have a sense of humor? What makes you a good partner, spouse, mother, sibling, friend, coworker, and so forth, and why?
- **Social status:** Do you have a good job, a nice car, or a beautiful apartment or house?
- **Appearance:** Do you like the way you dress or your shoes or your style? How do you feel about your height, weight, hair color, complexion, teeth, face, lips, eyes, mouth, chin, cheekbones, ears, nose, eyebrows, posture, shoulders, arms, shape of your hands, arms, legs, feet, and so forth?

Make a note of your answers to these questions, then draw your own self-esteem pie. Focus on your strengths first and leave the weaknesses and appearance items for last. Come up with as many pie slices as possible. It's a good idea to base your self-esteem on more than one or two areas, because it makes you less vulnerable. If you value perfect skin above anything else in yourself, even a tiny pimple can ruin your self-esteem, because you've nothing with which to balance it. However, if your skin is just one of many characteristics that factor into your self-evaluation, even a sunburn or multiple boils wouldn't rock your self-esteem in a major way. I hope you walked away from this exercise with a more balanced pie and a long list of qualities that can form the basis of your self-evaluation.

Modifying Negative Core Beliefs

In the preceding section, you learned how to broaden your perspective from a narrow appearance focus to seeing yourself and the world around you in a broader, more holistic way. Decreasing the importance of your appearance and basing your self-esteem on other aspects of your life will make you less vulnerable to body image concerns. In this section, you will learn how to address the more generalized negative core beliefs you may hold about yourself.

In Chapter 5, you learned about collecting the evidence for and against certain thoughts and interpretations you might have in your day-to-day life. Collecting the evidence is also a very powerful strategy when it comes to evaluating deeper-level core beliefs. Nadda initially believed very strongly that she was unlovable. The evidence that she used to support this belief was that her boyfriend had broken up with her. However, she then countered this evidence by realizing that the breakup also might have had something to do with her boyfriend's fear of commitment. Next she wrote down examples indicating that her old core belief, "I am unlovable," was not completely true. Thereafter, she reviewed all the evidence and summarized what she learned from this exercise. Finally, she developed a new belief that seemed better to fit the evidence she had collected. At the end of the exercise, she rated how much she believed her new belief; she also rerated her old belief. As you can see, her rating of the old belief dropped from 75% to 50% during the course of the exercise, and she even felt somewhat lovable. This was a pretty important discovery for Nadda. She kept working on collecting evidence supporting her lovability on her core belief records, and after 5 weeks her rating on her new belief that she was lovable had reached 80%!

Now you can go ahead and apply this strategy to yourself. However, beware that your new alternative belief shouldn't contain the word *not*, because you cannot define yourself in terms of what you are not, only in terms of who or what you are. For example, if your old belief was "I am ugly," a reasonable alternative belief might be "I look good enough" or "I look OK" rather than "I am not ugly." The new belief should also be plausible. A perfectionistic or usually positive core belief like "I look gorgeous" may be too strong for you to believe and therefore isn't likely to be useful either. Once you've found a plausible new core belief, you probably won't believe it 100% at first, because it is unfamiliar. Therefore, you'll have to keep working on it for some time. So, over the next few weeks, you might want to collect evidence that supports your new core belief and refutes your old one. Incorporate core belief records into your program several times a week.

How Should You Evaluate Your Progress?

I hope the exercises in this chapter have helped you modify your deeper-level beliefs and to reduce further the importance you give to your appearance imperfections. But if you aren't completely convinced yet that your old beliefs aren't true, don't worry. Keep in mind that a single application of the techniques described in this chapter is at best going to weaken core beliefs; it certainly

Core Belief Worksheet: Nadda

Old core belief: I'm unlovable.   *Strength of old belief*: 75%

Evidence that supports old core belief (try to counter it):

My boyfriend broke up with me. (But then, he's had so many girlfriends and never stays in relationships very long. His last girlfriend told me that he's commitment phobic.) So maybe this is something about him, not me ...

Evidence against this old core belief:

My mother and my siblings tell me that they love me.

When I recently had construction done on the house, my neighbors invited me to stay with them. They said I could come back anytime. They seem to like me.

At work many people stop by to chat for a few minutes, and sometimes my coworkers ask me for lunch. I guess they wouldn't do that if they didn't like me.

I have two very good friends. We've been close since we were kids and talk on the phone several times a week.

What I learned from this exercise:

I guess there are some people who like or even love me. Most of them have seen me one time or another in the past without makeup, and they still care about me. So I must be likable and lovable for reasons other than my appearance.

New core belief: I am likable and lovable.

Strength of new belief: 40%   *Strength of old belief*: 50%

Adapted by permission of the publisher and author from Judith S. Beck, *Cognitive Therapy: Basics and Beyond* (Guilford Press, © 1995).

Core Belief Worksheet

Old core belief: *Strength of old belief:*

Evidence that supports old core belief (try to counter it):

Evidence against this old core belief:

What I learned from this exercise:

New core belief:

Strength of new belief: *Strength of old belief:*

won't completely remove them. You've had these beliefs for a long time, and they'll likely shift only slowly. However, if you keep repeating these strategies, you'll find your old maladaptive beliefs will get weaker and your new beliefs will get stronger.

Over the next few weeks, you'll need to continue working on your Thought Records, ERP worksheets, and core belief records. Continue to conduct planned and systematic exercises for about 45 minutes to an hour per day, but also be flexible and address challenging situations as they come up. You know you've successfully completed this program when you've developed and strengthened healthier core beliefs, no longer avoid specific situations, and don't ritualize. So keep an eye on your self-monitoring logs and your ERP worksheets. Redo all the assessments from Chapter 4 about once a month and compare the goals you are currently working on with the long-term goals of the program. You know you're finished with the active phase of your program once you've reached all your long-term goals. At that point, you're ready for relapse prevention, which is described in Chapter 9.

Chapter 9

Staying Well

Over the last few weeks you've been working on progressively more challenging exercises. If your most recent assessment from Chapter 4 shows that you've reached all your long-term goals, congratulations! You can be very proud of what you've accomplished and are now ready to move on to relapse prevention. In this chapter, I'll show you how to move from the active phase of your program to the phase that's focused on staying well. Well-being is not a single event but a process. Lasting recovery requires certain skills that you can learn, like any other skill you've acquired so far. You can view the maintenance phase of your program as having three parts:

1. You start by tapering your practice time and reviewing the skills and insights that have helped you the most over the course of this program.
2. Then you learn how you can prevent relapse by recognizing and coping with high-risk situations.
3. Finally, you continue to take steps to lead a more balanced life by replacing rituals and avoidance with healthier habits.

Tapering Practice and Reviewing What You've Learned

After you've successfully completed the program in this book over approximately 12 weeks (keep in mind that you may take longer if your body image problems are more severe), it's important not to stop abruptly. Continue working on challenging situations as they come up while cutting in half the time you spend on scheduled exercise (such as completing Thought Records). If you feel ready, cut your practice down to every other day and keep reducing the frequency of your sessions over time. After you've done practice sessions every other day for 1 week, taper them to once a week, twice a month, once a month, once a season, and finally once a year. If you do well for the next couple of years, you can stop.

These intervals are just rough guidelines. If you start tapering your practice sessions and your body image problems start to come back, you may want to increase your practice session frequency again. You can always use the assessments in Chapter 4 to gauge whether your body image problems are returning if you're having trouble looking at this objectively.

Because your practice is less frequent, it can be easy to forget it altogether. To make sure you remember, mark your practice sessions on your calendar ahead of time.

The most important function of your practice sessions during this post-program period is to cement the gains you've made and arm yourself to deal with lapses effectively, so they don't become full-blown relapses. Toward that end, at the beginning of each practice session, review your progress using the worksheet on page 172 (make a generous number of copies of this form so that you have them on hand before each scheduled practice session):

Review the Strategies That Helped, the Insights Gained

Before you start tapering practice, review all the forms you completed over the course of your program and consider which strategies worked best for you during the program. You should have at least tried all the strategies described in Chapters 5–8, but many people find some of them more useful than others. It's extremely helpful to know which of the following strategies you can fall back on with the greatest degree of success:

- Reviewing your thinking errors and noting your most common ones (Chapter 5)
- Keeping Thought Records of negative thoughts, evaluating thoughts with questions to determine their usefulness (for example, "What are the advantages of this type of thinking?") and their validity (for example, "What is the evidence that this thought is really true?"), and generating rational alternatives to your thoughts (Chapter 5)
- Using exposure strategies (conducting planned exposures in situations you identified as challenging ahead of time, but also engaging in spontaneous ones when the opportunity presents itself) (Chapter 6):

    —evaluating your negative thoughts and developing rational alternatives to your original thoughts

Relapse Prevention Planning Worksheet

Date _____

How am I feeling?

How are my body image problems?

Did I attempt to complete my homework from the last practice? (If not, why not? What can I do to ensure that I am more successful with my homework next time?)

What skills/situations have I been working on successfully?

Where did I experience difficulties? What should I do about it?

What do I want to accomplish before my next practice session? What should my homework goals be?

Date for next practice session:

—setting specific goals that are realistic and within your control

—evaluating your efforts after the exposure and determining whether you achieved your goal and whether your negative thoughts came true, making a note of what you learned during the exercises

- Keeping track of your rituals and trying to reduce them as quickly as you can (Chapter 7), either by stopping cold turkey or by selecting one or a combination of these reduction methods:

—allowing rituals only in some situations, eliminating them in others

—decreasing the time or number of repetitions you allow for a particular ritual

—postponing the ritual to a later time

—using competing responses that are physically incompatible with the rituals or make it difficult for the ritual to occur

- Increasing healthy behaviors as you are decreasing rituals (Chapter 7)
- Learning to see the big picture when looking in the mirror (Chapter 7):

—describing your appearance objectively and nonjudgmentally

—avoiding any negative, emotionally charged labels for yourself

- Reducing comparisons of your own body parts of concern with those of others, noticing the big picture when you are with others (for example, the sound of their voices) (Chapter 7)
- Identifying self-defeating deeper-level beliefs (for example, with the downward arrow strategy)
- Broadening your perspective of your perceived appearance flaw to your other characteristics (Chapter 8) by

—writing a letter to your imagined children

—shifting your perspective by asking yourself what you respect in others

—asking yourself what kind of memories you want to have at the end of your life and how you want others to remember you at your funeral

—shifting your perspective from your perceived flaw to other aspects of yourself

—making a self-esteem pie that takes into account many areas of life (rather than just appearance)

- Modifying negative core beliefs by collecting evidence for–against old and new core beliefs

As you look through all your worksheets from the program, put a check mark next to the strategies in the preceding list that you found most effective. In addition to noting the treatment strategies that have worked well for you, pay attention to what you have learned over the course of the treatment. Fill out the worksheet on the following page and review the insights and strategies you listed during your practice sessions:

Relapse Prevention Review Worksheet

Strategies that worked best for me:

In what situations did these work well?

Why did they seem to work better than other strategies?

Most important insights:

Preventing Relapse

Toward the end of your program, you might be tempted to think you're done with practice and that your body image problems will never return again. But whether you've just finished your program or are at the point where you're practicing only once a year, there will be times when you'll experience urges to revert to your old appearance-related habits. These are especially likely to occur during periods of stress or distress. It's quite likely that you'll be able to maintain your gains and perhaps even improve more in the future, but you need to be prepared for temporary lapses during which you'll have to struggle to maintain your gains. First of all, don't overreact when a minor setback occurs. You'll have ups and downs, and that's completely normal. Just because you have days when you feel somewhat anxious about your looks or engage in some avoidance, comparing, or mirror checking doesn't mean that all your efforts were for nothing and you're now back to square one. A lapse should be taken as a sign that you need to practice a little more frequently the skills that helped you during the active phase of the program. A real relapse is different. It usually means you missed the early warning signs that you're slipping, and that your old problems are coming back. Fortunately, you can learn to prevent the high-risk situations and related lapses that may turn into a full-blown relapse.

Relapses often start during emotionally stressful situations. If you are well prepared for coping with those stressful situations, your chances for remaining well over the long term are high. Indeed, if you handle high-risk situations successfully, your perceived sense of control strengthens, which will make you less likely to relapse in the future. Success in coping with stressful situations will beget future success! If you expect to cope with a stressful situation successfully, you'll be less likely to give in to urges to ritualize and avoid.

To prevent relapse you'll have to learn to *recognize your own high-risk situations*. Try to think of something very stressful that might happen to you (for example, experiencing a personal rejection like a romantic breakup, losing a job, meeting someone who is unusually attractive, having your skin break out, getting a sunburn, scarring your skin, speaking to a group or doing something in a public setting, hearing family or friends comment on movie stars' or acquaintances' physical features, or having a family member become ill or die). Events that increase temptations to engage in beauty rituals should also be considered high-risk situations (for example, new media information about beauty products or cosmetic surgeries, or a friend telling you he or she is going to have cosmetic surgery). Then, in your mind, practice *coping with the high-risk situations*. Think about what you could do other than falling back into your negative thinking, rituals, or avoidance behaviors.

Practice your coping strategies through visualization. Your coping skills can include any of the strategies you have learned in treatment (for example, identifying problematic ways of thinking, practicing exposure or response prevention) or perhaps even enlisting the help of a support person. Refer to the Relapse Prevention Review Worksheet to remind yourself which strategies might work best in these imagined situations.

If you slip, limit the loss of control and watch out for negative self-talk, such as calling yourself a "hopeless loser" or a "total failure." Use your cognitive skills to detect and modify this version of all-or-nothing thinking. If you do have a setback (for example, if you had a skin-picking, hair-cutting, or avoidance episode), just admit you've made a mistake. Set the goal that you will limit the slip (such as to just one laser treatment, one declined invitation to go swimming) and/or call a support person when you have lost control. It might also help you to carry a "coping card" that lists responses to whatever negative thoughts you might have.

Scott, for example, called in sick at work because he had a pimple on his forehead. Although he initially felt relief that he didn't have to leave the house, thoughts about "wrecking all his efforts" and being "a wimp" and "a failure" crept in. His coping card read like this: "OK. This was a mistake; I should've gone to work. But people make mistakes, and lapses do occur. One mistake doesn't make me a total failure. I'll just learn from this experience and go to work tomorrow. I'll recommit myself to continued progress."

Later, he practiced handling his high-risk situation. He visualized how the following morning the pimple would still be there, and he would again have the urge to call in sick. But then he visualized that he would handle this situation well. He imagined himself completing a Thought Record with the following "Rational response": "My boss doesn't have perfect skin either. He doesn't pay me to work as a model but as a plumber. So it's really not that important what I look like!" He also visualized leaving the house and meeting his boss at work. He visualized that his eye contact would be good, despite the pimple. This visualization exercise helped him gain the confidence go to work the next day.

A More Balanced Lifestyle: Substituting Healthy Behaviors for Rituals and Avoidance

If you used to have very time-consuming beauty behaviors, it's important to think about what you can do with the extra time you gained by giving them up. It's important to fill this time in a meaningful way; otherwise the rituals will have a lot of room to creep back in to your routine. Similarly, you want to replace avoidance behaviors by participating in life more fully. You could either reengage in activities you used to do before your body image problems became such an issue or plan new activities. The possibilities are endless (for example, you could start a new hobby, such as painting or basketball; join a book club or dating service; find a volunteer or a paid job; go back to school or take a class for fun; start or join a support group or exercise class; learn how to play an instrument or how to meditate; start collecting stamps; play golf or soccer; go sailing, swimming, or horseback riding; play cards or other games; do needlepoint; go to the movies or to a play or a concert; do crossword or jigsaw puzzles; go out for coffee or dinner, or to a museum; go sight-seeing, hiking, or biking; go to a sauna, go skiing, or get involved in your community; or start getting massages). Most of your new activities should be social rather than solitary, so you can practice exposure to social situations without avoidance and giving in to beauty compulsions. Also keep in mind that if you want to increase your satisfaction in life, you might require a balance between some immediate pleasures (for example, going out for dinner with a friend) and long-term, meaningful goals that give you a sense of accomplishment or purpose (such as doing something that allows you to use your abilities or increase your spirituality).

Don't Give Up

Relapse prevention programs are usually successful, but you need to be prepared for the possibility that you'll have a relapse. Many people make the same New Year's resolutions for several years before they find the approach that works for them. Indeed, smokers often make three or more attempts to quit before they ultimately succeed. Relapses don't necessarily mean that you go back to where you started. You can learn from your mistakes, think of a better strategy, and build up your strength to try again. Try hard to prevent it, but if you do relapse, *don't give up*. Just try again!

Chapter 10

"Should I Take Medication?"

If you've already worked through the program in this book, you know that CBT techniques can be a significant amount of work. They are usually worth the effort, as many of the hundreds of patients I've treated would attest. Still, if you've struggled with this program, if you've had trouble preventing relapses, or if you're just having a bad day, you may wonder whether it would be easier and more effective just to take medication. For some people with BDD, medication can be quite helpful. But it's important to understand what medications can and cannot do, and to weigh the pros and cons before considering this approach to recovery. This chapter will give you a better idea about whether it would make sense for you to take medication, which medications and corresponding dosages may be effective, and what side effects you may experience. If you're interested in learning more, you will need to consult with a psychiatrist who has experience with BDD. (The Resources section of this book will provide you with suggestions for finding such a psychiatrist.)

The Pros and Cons of Medication

Medications can be very helpful for treating BDD and any accompanying symptoms of depression, which can be severe, and they may be lifesaving for people who are suicidal. If you have severe symptoms of depression, you may already be seeing a therapist and/or a psychiatrist; if you're not in therapy, ask your primary care physician for a referral, or use the guidelines I provide in the Resources section of this book to help you find a therapist.

Medications have advantages and disadvantages over cognitive-behavioral treatments. Among the advantages is that many patients consider taking medication easier than performing cognitive and behavioral exercises, which require more time and effort. Often, however, that time and effort pays off, as I said earlier. Because medications don't teach you any skills, there's a risk of relapse after medications are discontinued, especially if you discontinue the medications without having learned cognitive or behavioral skills first. Among the disadvantages of medications are potential side effects, although severe adverse effects are rare among the medications most commonly prescribed for body image concerns. The more typical mild to moderate side effects can often be managed successfully. The bottom line, in my opinion, is that medications are an option to consider, especially if cognitive and behavioral techniques haven't been sufficiently helpful. CBT and medication can work very well together—possibly better, in fact, than either treatment alone when BDD is severe.

"Shouldn't I Try to Resolve My Problems Myself, Rather Than Relying on Medications?"

Over the years I've met some people with rather extreme positions on medications, who either reject medications under any conditions or consider them the only solution. I encourage you to take a more moderate approach and evaluate all of your options for improvement. Remember that it is *not* a sign of weakness to ask for medications for your problems, any more than it would be to ask for medical help for heart disease, diabetes, or an infection. Indeed, treating your body image problems in the best possible way is the most responsible thing to do.

"When *Is* It Appropriate to Consider Medication?"

If the cognitive and behavioral exercises described in this book aren't working or you're having trouble completing even the lowest-ranked items on your avoidance hierarchy, adding medication might be an appropriate solution. Keep in mind that everyone responds differently to treatment. You just have to find the treatment, or the combination of treatments that work for you.

Alan had severe BDD. He was completely convinced that he looked ugly and that others were constantly staring at or mocking his long nose. He only rarely left the house because he felt highly anxious in social situations, and he often asked his mother to go food shopping or do other errands for him. He kept touching his nose and asked for reassurance from his parents many times a day. He had stopped working as an engineer several years before coming to our clinic, because he thought his coworkers were laughing at him. When he came to our program, he initially wanted to try only CBT. However, because of his high degree of conviction about his ugliness, he had difficulty coming up with rational responses in Thought Records. Due to his high anxiety (even around me), he was unable to complete any exposure exercises or to control his compulsive behavior. Therefore, I broached the subject of medication with him. After a discussion of the pros and cons of medication, Alan agreed to meet with a psychiatrist. After about 6 weeks on fluvoxamine (Luvox), his condition began to improve dramatically. His anxiety, compulsions, and avoidance behavior decreased. Overall, his symptoms improved by about 40%. Although this was a substantial improvement, some symptoms remained. When he tried CBT again (he was still taking fluvoxamine), Alan was able to reduce his symptoms even further. He has now been on medication for 2 years. His BDD symptoms are pretty minimal, and he has started to work again.

The more severe your body image concerns, the more distress they will cause you and, in turn, the greater their interference with your life. The more severe your symptoms are, then, the more seriously you should consider a combination of CBT and medication. This is especially true if you have not only body image concerns but also other problems such as depression. In general, we tend to prescribe appropriate medications to anyone who requests this type of treatment in our clinic. However, if you are pregnant or breast-feeding, you should take medication only after a careful review of the pros and cons and a consultation with a physician experienced with the effects of such medications on pregnancy and nursing.

Medication Treatments for BDD

Over the last decade, we have learned a lot about medication treatment for BDD. Serotonin reuptake inhibitors (SRIs) are the medications most frequently prescribed for treating BDD, and they appear to be at least partially effective for the majority of patients. They have even demonstrated effectiveness in treating people with very low-insight and delusional BDD. SRIs include clomipramine (Anafranil) and a similar class of medications called *selective serotonin reuptake inhibitors* (SSRIs). The SSRIs act on the serotonin system more specifically than does clomipramine, which also affects other neurotransmitters. Serotonin is one of the chemical messengers between brain cells. The SRIs increase the amount of serotonin between nerve cells by preventing its reuptake into the releasing nerve cell. Therefore, more serotonin is available between nerve cells, which likely increases the availability of serotonin to important areas of the brain. The SRIs appear to correct a chemical imbalance in the brain, and patients often describe feeling more normal when taking them. As a group, the SSRIs are safe medications. They won't create an artificial state of happiness, and they are not addictive.

Of the several studies conducted on SRIs in BDD, the best studies so far were two double-blind, randomized, controlled trials. *Randomized* means that the patients were randomly assigned to receive either a particular medication or a placebo (sugar pill); *double-blind* means that neither the patient nor the doctor knew which medication the patient was receiving; and *controlled* means that the active drug was compared with something else, either a placebo or another medication, rather than with nothing at all. In the first of those double-blind, randomized, controlled trials, Dr. Eric Hollander found that clomipramine was more effective than the non-SRI antidepressant desipramine for BDD symptoms. The other study was conducted by Dr. Katharine Phillips, who found that fluoxetine (Prozac) was significantly more effective than placebo (sugar pill) in treating patients with BDD symptoms. In addition to these studies, several studies that did not include a comparison group were conducted; these studies showed that the SSRIs citalopram (Celexa), escitalopram (Lexapro), and fluvoxamine (Luvox) reduced BDD symptoms for most patients.

"What's the Right Dose?"

The different SRIs tend to be most effective at different doses.

Typically, patients who suffer from BDD require dosages at the higher end of the therapeutic range for SRIs, and the typical doses for BDD are higher than for other disorders, such as depression. Before switching to a different drug, the highest recommended dosage for a given SRI should be tried, as long as the drug is tolerated. If your dose is not high enough, your symptoms might improve only slightly or not at all.

In her book *The Broken Mirror*, Dr. Phillips recommends that the dosage be raised fairly quickly to reach the maximum dose recommended within 4–9 weeks from the beginning of treatment, as long as side effects aren't a problem. The advantage of increasing the dose quickly is that you'll probably respond faster to treatment than if the dose is increased slowly.

Medication	Typical daily dose range (mg) for depression	Average daily dose (mg) and standard deviation* for patients with BDD
Citalopram (Celexa)	20–60	66 ± 36
Escitalopram (Lexapro)	10–30	29 ± 12
Fluvoxamine (Luvox)	100–300	308 ± 49
Fluoxetine (Prozac)	20–80	67 ± 24
Paroxetine (Paxil)	20–60	55 ± 13
Sertraline (Zoloft)	50–200	202 ± 46
Clomipramine (Anafranil)	100–250	203 ± 53

Adapted by permission of the publisher and author from Katharine A. Phillips, *The Broken Mirror: Understanding and Treating Body Dysmorphic Disorder* (Oxford University Press, © 1996, 2005).
*Standard deviations indicate the range of doses used for about two thirds of patients with BDD in Dr. Phillips's clinical sample. For instance, for fluvoxamine, about two thirds of patients received between 259 mg per day and 357 mg per day.

"Which SRI Might Be Right for Me?"

All SRIs seem to be effective for BDD, even for patients who have very low insight or are delusional, so you can start with any one of them. As I described earlier, some of the SRIs have been studied more extensively, but clinical experience shows that all of them may be helpful. If one doesn't work for you, another one may work and is worth trying. Because the SSRIs have fewer side effects than clomipramine, it is common to start with one of those medications. However, if you don't respond to one or more of the SSRIs, clomipramine is worth trying. Clomipramine should not be prescribed in doses exceeding 250mg per day, because more severe side effects (for example, seizures) can occur in this higher range.

"What Side Effects Do the SRIs Have?"

People who take clomipramine may experience dry mouth, constipation, light-headedness, and blurred vision, especially at higher doses. SSRIs may cause nausea, headaches, disturbed sleeping patterns, and occasionally increased anxiety (although anxiety symptoms more typically improve). However, these side effects often disappear within a couple of weeks. SSRIs and clomipramine can lead to changes in weight or sexual difficulties (for example, decreased sex drive or inability to experience an orgasm, difficulties that go away when the medication is stopped).

"Can the Side Effects Be Managed?"

It's important to realize that side effects can often be managed very easily. For example, if you have nausea, you might be able to relieve this problem by taking your medication with meals. If your sleep patterns are disrupted because of the medication, you might want to take the medication at a different time of the day. If you have problems with your libido, your dose might be lowered, or you might be prescribed an additional medication. On the other hand, if the side effects are severe, you might have to switch to another SRI. The rule of thumb is that the side effects should never be worse than the problem for which they were prescribed.

   If you do have side effects, be sure to discuss them with your prescribing physician so that you can develop a strategy to manage them.

"How Long Will It Take for the Medication to Work?"

Be patient. It might take several weeks for a medication to start working, so it's important that you try the SRI for a sufficient amount of time. To get an adequate trial of an SRI, you should take it for 12–16 weeks; a higher dosage may be needed if your symptoms don't improve with a lower dose. Most likely your SRI will not change your symptoms overnight; rather, your BDD symptoms will improve gradually. Unfortunately, no research so far has examined whether CBT makes medications work faster, but based on my clinical experience, I certainly believe that it does.

"Should I Take the Medication Only on Days When I Feel Bad?"

It's extremely important that you take your medication each and every day, exactly as prescribed by your clinician. If your take a lower dose than your doctor recommends, or if you take your medication irregularly, you may not benefit from your treatment. Also, even if you start to feel better while taking the medication, don't discontinue it, or skip or lower your doses. This could result in a recurrence of your symptoms. If you think your dose too high or too low, be sure to tell your doctor, who can adjust your medication dosage, if necessary.

"If the Medication Works, How Long Should I Stay on It?"

Most likely you will continue to feel better as long as you take your medication. But you might wonder how long you should stay on the medication if your body image symptoms improve. Unfortunately, we have no data to answer this question, although at the time of publication, Dr. Phillips and I were doing a research study to answer this important question. As far as we know, the SRIs don't have any long-term, irreversible side effects. Patients who have had very severe BDD often stay on them for many years without difficulties. This is probably a good idea, because symptoms may return after an effective SSRI is discontinued. However, if you plan on becoming pregnant, or if your side effects are more severe than the benefits you derive from the medications, you should have a discussion with your doctor about the pros and cons of staying on the medication. Most patients seem to stay on the medication for at least 1 or 2 years, even if they are feeling better. However, at some point, many people want to discontinue an efficacious SRI, because the alternative is lifelong treatment.

Consider Alan, who was doing well with a combination of medication and CBT. He stopped CBT after 4 months of successful weekly sessions and was taking a stable dose of medication for a total of 2 years. The combination treatment helped him greatly; he performed well at his job, started socializing more, and began dating and enjoying his life. Nevertheless, he had some mild sexual side effects while taking the medication; therefore, Alan wanted to see how he would do without it. He and his psychiatrist worked out a plan for decreasing his dosage very slowly over the course of 1 year. Despite this slow taper, some of his BDD symptoms recurred during the medication discontinuation phase. For example, he was more anxious when someone was looking directly at him, and he began to avoid eye contact in those situations. He also started checking the mirror occasionally and asking for reassurance regarding his appearance. When he noticed that some of his symptoms returned, he and his doctor decided that he should start his CBT sessions again (another option would have been to increase the medication). Currently, Alan is doing well. He is not taking any medications, and he attends monthly CBT treatment sessions to prevent relapse.

If you do choose to go off the medication, discuss this with your clinician and taper it slowly. Also, try to taper the medication at a time when you don't have too many stressors in your life. For example, it's not a good idea to stop a medication right after losing your job. In my clinical experience, patients who have received CBT appear to be more likely to taper without relapse. The cognitive and behavioral techniques seem to enable them to control the symptoms that may return when they stop taking medications.

"If the Medication Doesn't Work, What Can I Do?"

If you start taking a medication and don't respond to it, or respond only minimally, you and your physician need to determine whether you have been on the medication long enough and at a high enough dose. If you have, your physician might recommend that you switch to another SRI. Another option might be to add a second medication to improve the effectiveness of the original medication. This strategy, called *augmentation*, seems particularly useful when someone has responded partially (rather than not at all) to the first medication. In *The Broken Mirror*, Dr. Katharine A. Phillips suggests a number of different augmentors, including the atypical neuroleptics (especially Geodon, but also Zyprexa, or Risperdal), the antianxiety medication buspirone (BuSpar), and the antidepressant venlafaxine (Effexor). She also mentions that occasionally patients respond to lithium, methylphenidate (Ritalin), or bupropion (Wellbutrin), or other medications. Additional treatment with benzodiazepines should be considered when patients are very anxious or distressed. To learn more about these medications or pharmacotherapy for treatment of BDD in general, I suggest you read Chapter 13 in *The Broken Mirror* (see Resources).

Since most of this book is devoted to CBT, you've probably already tried the cognitive and behavioral exercises. However, if you started out with medication and it did not work adequately for you, I strongly encourage you to try cognitive and behavioral strategies. Depending on the severity of your problem, you might do this either by yourself, with the help of this book, or under the supervision of a trained cognitive-behavioral therapist. Of course, as I described earlier, you can also start CBT and medication at the same time, since they may work well together.

Chapter 11

Helping a Family Member
or Friend
with Body Image Concerns

People who have body image problems experience considerable pain, but they are not the only ones who suffer. Family members and friends are also affected. If you have a relative or friend with a body image disturbance or BDD, this chapter is for you. If you are the person with the body image concerns, you might want to read this chapter to gain an understanding of how your problem is affecting those who care about you. Sometimes knowing that you're not the only one feeling pain over your concerns about how you look provides just the extra nudge you need to seek help and try to change. But if you are already working through the program, you don't need to read this chapter.

If someone you care about is so wrapped up in appearance concerns that life has become circumscribed and unrewarding, and you're worried about the person's future, you know what a tough dilemma this can be. How can you expect people to understand why your spouse or child is never seen anywhere? Your colleagues might wonder if he or she even exists. How do you explain the last-minute excuses made to bow out of attending a party or other social event? It can be embarrassing to keep making excuses for a family member, trying to cover up what may look like a lack of interest or bad manners. It can also be frus-

and over again if his hair looks all right? How should you react if your daughter tells you that she will feel better only if she has plastic surgery?

Like any other illness, BDD can take a toll on the family members and friends of the sufferer. If someone you love has BDD, you'll probably experience confusion, fear, anger, and guilt. It's very difficult to watch someone you care about suffer, and you might feel unsure of how to help. This chapter will give you some guidance for what you can do for a friend or relative with BDD or body image concerns that are severe enough to interfere significantly with his or her life—and yours, without sacrificing your own well-being.

Learn about the Problem

You may feel confused about why your loved one ended up with this problem, how to approach this person, and how to get help. The best first step toward answering these questions is to educate yourself about BDD. Read this book and check out the Resources section at the end of the book. You might even want to talk to a professional who knows about BDD. Educating yourself will help you understand what to expect from the person you know who has BDD, and from the recovery process.

Tell Your Relative or Friend about This Program

After you've educated yourself about BDD, approach the person privately. Ensure that you don't get interrupted and leave plenty of time to discuss the issue. Tell your friend or relative about the symptoms you noticed, and be as direct and specific as you can (for example, "It seems to me that you think and talk a lot about your nose. You also spend a lot of time in front of the mirror, and lately you've always declined when I asked you to come to any social events. You seem so anxious and unhappy. I'm really worried about you!") Say that you're concerned that he or she might have a body image problem called *body dysmorphic disorder*. Listen to what the person has to say, ask questions, and don't judge. Tell your friend or relative that you'd like to help him or her feel better. Present the person with the information you've gathered (for example, from this book and other resources). Then try to engage the person in a discussion about what to do next. Perhaps he or she would like to try the self-help approach described in earlier chapters. In this case, offer to act as a support person. If the problem seems severe according to the assessment in Chapter 4, ask the person to make an appointment with a professional who knows about BDD to get an appropriate diagnosis and treatment.

Be Supportive: Offer to Be a Helper

Your social support is critical to the person with BDD. He or she needs your understanding, patience, and encouragement. Do not belittle the negative feelings he or she expresses; offer hope. Suggest that you and the affected person work on the different steps outlined in this book together. Complete Thought Records and help your relative think of exposure exercises, such as movies, walks, and other outings. Help him or her set realistic goals for response prevention. Also ask what he or she would like you to do if you catch him or her in the middle of a BDD ritual. Agree on ways in which you could help with interrupting those rituals. Perhaps your loved one will suggest that you make certain statements as reminders of the big picture (for example, "Are your eyebrows really more important than your aunt's funeral right now? How likely is it that people will be thinking about your eyebrows at this event?").

If your relative has given up many activities he or she enjoyed in the past, encourage him or her to restart those activities. Pushing too hard, however, is likely to overwhelm and discourage your relative, so take it slowly. When helping someone with BDD, it's important to maintain a positive outlook. People with BDD have low self-esteem and need to know that you care about them and believe in their ability to overcome this problem. Encourage your relative to stay with the self-help program described in this book until the symptoms improve (which will take several weeks or months), even if it causes a high level of anxiety, or if a particular exercise is a real struggle.

As I mentioned earlier, if your loved one's symptoms are too severe to be treated via self-help, encourage him or her to make an appointment with a licensed psychologist, psychiatrist, or social worker who specializes in treatment of BDD. If your relative or friend is hesitant to go to the first few appointments alone, offer to go along.

If the first treatment approach does not work, encourage your friend to seek alternatives. If multiple outpatient treatments produce limited success and/or if the problem is severe, suggest residential treatment programs that specialize in BDD (see the Resources section at the back of the book for specific recommendations).

Seek Emergency Care If Necessary

Don't ignore remarks about suicide. **If your loved one is suicidal, get professional help immediately.** Contact the nearest emergency room or the person's mental health provider.

Don't Enable

Don't enable a person with body image concerns. As I mentioned earlier, you don't want to force the person, which might lead to major conflicts, but don't let him or her off the hook too easily if the person avoids facing his or her fears. Always encourage the person to take one additional step when he or she is tempted to avoid something. Don't agree to participate in compulsive or avoidance behaviors, whether it's paying for cosmetic surgery or driving the person to BDD-related dermatologists' visits. This can be challenging, because the affected person might get angry if you don't participate in rituals. Keep in mind that you are helping your loved one much more by not enabling those behaviors.

Try to come to an agreement ahead of time as to how you'll handle specific BDD-related behaviors and be reasonably firm when setting limits. Sometimes you might have to fade out your participation in BDD rituals gradually; in this case, you will negotiate how many repetitions of a particular ritual per day are OK. For example, if your loved one asks: "How does my hair look?" You might respond, "Honey, we've agreed that I will answer these kinds of questions only once a day, and I've already answered this morning, so I'm not going to respond right now." If the person gets extremely angry or upset when you refuse to participate in rituals, accompany him or her to a therapist to develop a plan for dealing with the specific BDD behaviors, as well as the conflicts that arise as a result of BDD.

Maintain a Normal Routine and Don't Sacrifice Your Own Happiness

Don't let the person with BDD disrupt the entire household. Your family should maintain its normal routine as much as possible. If you sacrifice your own activities too often, you might ultimately end up resenting the person with BDD. If something is important to you, and you can't get the person to do it with you, learn to do things independently. Keep in mind that no matter how much you love this person, there's a limit to what you can and should do. Trying to help someone with BDD can be emotionally draining, and the recovery process might be long. Therefore, keep recharging your own batteries. Do something nice for yourself every day. See friends or take a job that takes you out of the house, or read a good book.

If you are very distressed about the issues that go along with having a family member with BDD, you might want to seek help for yourself. Make an appointment with a therapist to get some guidance for dealing with the feelings you are experiencing. If there's a support group in your area for families who have a member with mental illness, you might want to think about joining it. If there is none, you could start one. Keep in mind that by taking good care of your own well-being, you'll be emotionally stronger and therefore in a better position to help your friend or family member with BDD. Remind yourself that you deserve to enjoy life even if your loved one is not able to do so.

Don't Get Angry

At times you might feel angry toward the person with BDD if he or she claims not to have the disorder (claiming instead to have a physical defect). Your relative or friend might also push your buttons with repeated avoidance behaviors and endless appearance rituals. Keep in mind that this behavior isn't aimed at you personally or intended to hurt you. It comes from having a true mental disorder. Having an illness is not a character flaw, and is nobody's fault.

Don't argue with the person about whether he or she has BDD or whether the perceived defect is real or imagined. Yelling will likely not improve the situation and will only cause the person to feel worse. This might reinforce beliefs about inadequacy and worthlessness, which in turn might lead to more BDD behaviors. Instead, be compassionate and emphasize that you are concerned because you see your loved one suffering. Remind the person that you don't think that he or she will start to feel better without an intervention.

Be prepared for the possibility that your friend or family member will refuse to seek help, which can be very frustrating. Keep in mind you cannot force someone into a self-help program or other treatment. You can only express your concerns and observations. Remember that you can bring up the subject again in the future, and do it!

If you're frustrated, keeping your frustration inside is not a useful strategy, so try to talk to someone about it. You can talk to friends, a therapist, or member of the clergy, or, as I suggested earlier, you can join a support group for families.

Don't Feel Guilty

Many people, especially parents, find themselves feeling guilty because they somehow feel responsible for their family member's developing BDD. You might also feel guilty because you couldn't prevent the problem, or because you don't have a magic cure. Blaming yourself will not help anyone; it will only make you feel worse. It's more useful to accept the fact that there is a problem and begin working toward helping the person and yourself. Examine the beliefs underlying your guilt and, if appropriate, use the techniques from Chapter 5 to evaluate those beliefs. For example, if you think, "I never should have said this to her," read or reread Chapter 2 of this book, which describes the likely causes of body image concerns, and remind yourself that one single negative comment is not going to cause BDD. Many factors have to come together to enable body image problems to develop. Don't dwell on the past and what you have or haven't done. You can't change it anyway. Focus on how to improve the current situation and the future for yourself and your loved ones.

Recognize Small Accomplishments and Keep Your Expectations Realistic

Realize that there's no magic cure for BDD, and there aren't any quick solutions. Demanding change or berating your family member about not improving fast enough will not be fruitful. Educate yourself about the treatment process; this will help you keep your expectations realistic. Whether the person is using the self-help approach described in this book, seeing a therapist, or taking medication (or a combination of these methods), it's likely to take months to change the negative thoughts, avoidance patterns, and beauty rituals. Expect progress to have ups and downs, so avoid day-to-day comparisons. Recognize achievements even if they are small. Be patient; over time your loved one will attempt more and more difficult goals. Let your relative know when he or she has done a good job, and if the person can complete only part of a goal, praise him or her anyway. This will help the person with BDD keep going.

There Is Hope

Never forget that BDD can be overcome. During the recovery process, your loved one will experience lapses, but that's normal. Don't be discouraged; no one can recover from this overnight. It may take time and effort, but BDD can be beaten.

Appendix

The Relationship of BDD to Other Disorders

Several other disorders can look like BDD, and they can also coexist with it. If you think you may have one of these disorders instead of or along with BDD, however, only a qualified professional can make an accurate diagnosis and provide the appropriate treatment. The following is intended solely as a general indicator of whether you should consult a mental health practitioners to obtain a diagnosis and treatment.

The figures on the rate of co-occurrence with BDD all come from research by Dr. Katharine Phillips.

Eating Disorders

- *Similarities with BDD*: Excessive focus on appearance; distorted body image (those with anorexia nervosa usually view themselves as "fat" when they are in fact emaciated); repetitive behaviors such as mirror checking and body measuring; hiding certain body parts (for example, thighs) out of shame; overexercising and changes in eating behavior.

- *Differences from BDD*: Patients with anorexia are concerned that, overall, they are too fat, or could get fat, whereas the focus in BDD is usually on specific features or body parts, such as the nose. Patients with anorexia look very abnormal (that is, much too thin), whereas BDD patients look normal (as do many bulimia nervosa patients, who tend to maintain weight in the normal range). BDD sufferers may change eating patterns occasionally to change the appearance of a specific body part (for example, they might diet to change the appearance of a round chin), but they don't engage in disturbed eating patterns consistently and for the general purpose of losing weight. Patients with BDD don't usually purge (via laxatives or vomiting) or binge (as in bulimia).

Nevertheless, there's a gray zone between BDD and eating disorders. I usually diagnose a person who has excessive concerns about "fat thighs" but not overall body weight and doesn't have disturbed eating habits, for example, with BDD. However, some researchers would disagree with this.

About 12% of persons with BDD also have an eating disorder.

If you have symptoms of both BDD and an eating disorder, you must learn to gain control over your eating behavior, and this usually needs to be done with the help of a mental health professional who specializes in eating disorders.

Obsessive–Compulsive Disorder

• *Similarities with BDD*: Preoccupations with particular ideas (obsessions) and ritualistic behaviors (compulsions).

• *Differences from BDD*: In BDD, the obsessions and compulsions are restricted to concerns about appearance.

About 25% of persons with BDD also have obsessive–compulsive disorder.

Obsessive–compulsive disorder requires specialized treatment. There are some very good self-help books (for example, *Getting Control* by Dr. Lee Baer, *Mastery of Obsessive–Compulsive Disorder* by Drs. Edna Foa and Michael Kozak, or *Overcoming Obsessive–Compulsive Disorder Client Manual* by Dr. Gail Steketee), but severe symptoms require the treatment of a mental health professional.

Social Phobia

• *Similarities with BDD*: Self-consciousness in and avoidance of social situations.

• *Differences from BDD*: Social anxiety usually focuses on particular situations, commonly public speaking, eating in restaurants, taking tests, writing in public, using public restrooms, dating, and stage fright (for example, entertaining an audience). People with social phobia don't focus on their appearance or have the desire to fix their appearance with the rituals described in this chapter.

About 32% of patients with BDD also suffer from social phobia.

Many of the exercises in this book can be applied easily to all forms of social anxiety. If your social phobia symptoms are mild, also consider the self-help books by Drs. Martin M. Antony and Richard Swinson (*The Shyness and Social Anxiety Workbook*) or Dr. Debra Hope and colleagues (*Managing Social Anxiety*). For more severe problems, seek consultation with a cognitive-behavioral therapist or a psychopharmacologist.

Depression

- *Similarities with BDD*: People with depression often think they are unattractive; people with severe appearance concerns are often depressed.

- *Differences from BDD*: Those who suffer from depression have other problems besides being concerned about their looks—feeling sad or irritable most of the day; losing interest in things they once considered important and enjoyable; having difficulty sleeping; feeling worthless or guilty; having difficulty concentrating, having no appetite; and, in severe cases, having thoughts of suicide.

Three quarters of patients with BDD are also depressed. There are several explanations for this high rate of co-occurrence:

1. Negative thinking—if you discount all the great qualities you have and focus instead on just one imperfection, you are more likely to feel hopeless.
2. Avoidance behavior related to your appearance concerns can also cause or contribute to depression by making you feel lonely and feel that your life is restricted.

If your depression is mild and directly related to your appearance concerns, the symptoms of depression might improve as a result of this program. However, severe depression requires more than just reading this book. If you think you fit the criteria for depression, please seek professional help. *If you have thoughts about suicide, you need to seek emergency care immediately.*

Trichotillomania

- *Similarities with BDD*: Hair pulling (from the scalp, eyelashes, eyebrows, or other parts of the body), resulting in noticeable bald patches; avoidance behavior (for example, those with trichotillomania may not put their head under water while swimming and might cover missing hair with hairpieces or hairstyles, scarves, clothing, or makeup).

- *Differences from BDD*: In BDD, hair pulling is done to improve appearance; in trichotillomania it is done in response to an impulse.

Only 2% of persons with BDD also have trichotillomania. But (from a study by Jennifer Soriano at Massachusetts General Hospital), 26% of patients with trichotillomania also have BDD.

For mild to moderate trichotillomania, the book *Help for Hair Pullers* by Dr. Nancy Keuthen and colleagues might be helpful. For severe trichotillomania, meet with a cognitive behavior therapist or a psychopharmacologist.

Resources

Finding a Clinician

If your BDD symptoms are severe or didn't fully respond to the self-help approach described in this book, consider making an appointment with a mental health treatment provider. Most likely, you'll have to look around a little before you find a qualified clinician. Although we know that BDD can be treated successfully with certain cognitive behavioral strategies, not all therapists are familiar with these techniques, and even fewer are familiar with BDD. Therefore, before you agree to start treatment with a particular therapist, ask the clinician to describe his or her treatment approach to you. This description should list some of the cognitive strategies described earlier in this book (for example, the identification and subsequent modification of self-defeating thoughts) as well as exposure and response prevention. If the therapist is knowledgeable about cognitive and behavioral approaches in general but is not familiar with BDD, ask whether he or she has treated obsessive–compulsive disorder or social phobia (the treatment of these disorders is similar to CBT for BDD). If so, this therapist should have at least a basic knowledge of the critical elements for treating BDD, and perhaps you might suggest using this book to tailor the treatment to your body image problems.

If you've decided you want to consider taking medication, try to find a licensed psychiatrist who is experienced with psychopharmacology for BDD (or if you can't find one who has experience with BDD, try to find one who is familiar with obsessive–compulsive disorder).

If you live near a major university or medical school, you might start by calling its psychology or psychiatry department and asking for a clinician with experience in BDD. Or ask your primary care physician for a referral. If this does not provide any leads, check out the organizations and websites listed in the following pages, many of which will provide you with information on BDD and/or help you find a therapist or psychopharmacologist.

Specialty Clinics

Body Dysmorphic Disorder Clinic and Research Unit
Massachusetts General Hospital and Harvard Medical School
Simches Research Building
185 Cambridge Street
Boston, MA 02114
Phone: 617-726-6766
Website: www.massgeneral.org/bdd/

This clinic that I founded in 1998 offers the treatment program on which this book is based, as well as serving as a research unit. The website provides information about BDD and the different outpatient treatment options available at this program, as well as a listing of ongoing studies. Treatment is free of charge for individuals who qualify for treatment studies. The resources page on the website lists national mental health organizations with a broader focus, which might be of help to you, in addition to the BDD-focused organizations below.

Body Image Program
Butler Hospital
345 Blackstone Boulevard
Providence, RI 02906
Phone: 401-455-6200
Websites: www.bodyimageprogram.com; www.butler.org/body.cfm?id=123

This large BDD outpatient treatment program is headed by BDD expert Dr. Katharine Phillips. The website has listings of free treatment studies, as well as a comprehensive listing of treatment providers around the world.

Compulsive, Impulsive, and Anxiety Disorders Program
Mount Sinai School of Medicine
One Gustave L. Levy Place
P.O. Box 1230
New York, NY 10029
Phone: 917-492-9449
Website: www.mssm.edu/psychiatry/ciadp/index.shtml

The program specializes in the outpatient treatment of obsessive–compulsive disorder, BDD, and related disorders, and offers free treatment studies for BDD to eligible patients. Dr. Eric Hollander, who heads this program, and Dr. Andrea Allen are internationally recognized BDD experts.

Biobehavioral Institute
935 Northern Boulevard
Great Neck, NY 11021
Phone: 516-487-7116
Website: www.bio-behavioral.com/home.asp

The Biobehavioral Institute specializes in the outpatient treatment of obsessive–compulsive disorder, BDD, and related disorders. The clinical services of this program are directed by Dr. Fugen Neziroglu, who has published extensively on BDD. The website provides helpful information for people with BDD.

UCLA Anxiety Disorders Program
Phone: 310-206-5133
Website: www.semel.ucla.edu/adc/index.html

The UCLA Anxiety Disorders Program provides treatment for BDD, as well as the opportunity to participate in BDD research studies.

Los Angeles Body Dysmorphic Disorder Clinic
10850 Wilshire Boulevard, Suite 240
Los Angeles, CA 90024
Phone: 310-741-2000
E-mail: director@bddclinic.com
Website: www.bddclinic.com

The Los Angeles Body Dysmorphic Disorder Clinic is the first mental health clinic on the west coast of the United States dedicated primarily to the evaluation and treatment of BDD. The clinical staff specialize in the treatment of BDD as well as other psychiatric disorders that frequently co-exist with it.

Obsessive–Compulsive Disorders Institute at McLean Hospital
115 Mill Street
Belmont, MA 02478
Phone: 617-855-3279
Website: www.mclean.harvard.edu/patient/adult/ocd.php

The Obsessive–Compulsive Disorders Institute is a residential treatment program for individuals ages 16 and older. It predominantly specializes in the treatment of obsessive–compulsive disorder but it also treats individuals with BDD.

Menninger Clinic
2801 Gessner Drive
P.O. Box 809045
Houston, TX 77280
Phone: 800-351-9058
Website: www.menningerclinic.com/p-ocd/index.htm

The Menninger Obsessive–Compulsive Disorders Treatment Program provides an inpatient treatment program for adolescents ages 12–17, and a program for adults, ages 18 and older, who have severe obsessive–compulsive disorder, BDD, or related disorders. This program specializes in individuals who need extensive staff support and/or have been in outpatient treatment without the desired success.

Rogers Memorial Hospital
Obsessive–Compulsive Disorder Center
34700 Valley Road
Oconomowoc, WI 53066
Phone: 800-767-4411
Website: www.rogershospital.org/obsessive_compulsivedisorders.php

The Obsessive–Compulsive Disorder Center provides intensive treatment for severe obsessive–compulsive disorder and related disorders, including BDD. It offers a residential treatment program as well as a partial hospitalization program.

BDD Treatment Programme
The Priory Hospital North London
Grovelands House
Southgate
London N14 6RA, United Kingdom
Phone: 020 8882 8191
Website: www.veale.co.uk/appoint.html#treatment

The Priory Hospital in London offers inpatient, day-patient, or outpatient treatment programs for adolescents and adults with obsessive–compulsive disorder or BDD. Call to make an appointment with the internationally recognized BDD expert Dr. David Veale or his staff members.

Centre for Anxiety Disorders and Trauma
99 Denmark Hill
London SE5 8AF, United Kingdom
Phone: 0207 919 2101; 0207 919 3286
E-mail: anxietydisordersunit@slam.nhs.uk

Websites: psychology.iop.kcl.ac.uk/cadat/patients/BDD.aspx; www.veale.co.uk/maudsley.html

This British organization provides treatment for BDD and also maintains a website that offers information on BDD, as well as a listing of research studies on BDD.

Organizations and Websites

BDD Central
Website: www.bddcentral.com

This comprehensive website provides general education about BDD, as well as a list of mental health professionals from the United States and abroad who have experience with the treatment of BDD. It also lists extensive resources and links to many BDD-related websites.

Obsessive–Compulsive Foundation
676 State Street
New Haven, CT 06511
Phone: 203-401-2070
E-mail: info@ocfoundation.org
Website: www.ocfoundation.org

This foundation has a website providing information about obsessive–compulsive disorder and related disorders (including BDD). The foundation's mission is to provide assistance to individuals with obsessive–compulsive disorder and related disorders, which includes BDD, and to support research on treatments for those disorders. It publishes a newsletter and sponsors an annual conference for patients that regularly includes presentations about BDD. It has an international treatment provider list. In addition to helping you find treatment, the foundation can help if you would like to start a BDD support group.

Association for Behavioral and Cognitive Therapies
305 Seventh Avenue, 16th floor
New York, NY 10001-6008
Phone: 212-647-1890
Website: www.aabt.org/

Formerly the Association for Advancement of Behavior Therapy, this group can help with a referral to a CBT therapist. Its website allows you to search for a therapist by state and certain search criteria (it doesn't list BDD specifically, but you can search for social anxiety or obsessive–compulsive disorder).

Academy of Cognitive Therapy (ACT)
One Belmont Avenue, Suite 700
Bala Cynwyd, PA 19004-1610
Phone: 610-664-1273
Fax: 610-664-5137
E-mail: info@academyofct.org
Website: www.academyofct.org

The ACT is a nonprofit organization that supports and furthers research in cognitive therapy. Its website provides a list of certified cognitive therapies in 31 different countries as well as information on several mental health disorders, research in the field, and information on cognitive therapy.

British Association for Behavioural and Cognitive Psychotherapies
The Globe Centre
P.O. Box 9
Accrington BB5 0XB, United Kingdom
Phone: 01254 875277
Website: www.babcp.com/

This association can provide you with a referral for a cognitive-behavioral therapist.

OCD Action
22/24 Highbury Grove, Suite 107
London N5 2EA, United Kingdom
Phone: 0845 390 6232
Website: www.ocdaction.org.uk

This British organization aimed mainly at obsessive–compulsive disorder also offers a variety of resources for BDD, including a list of support groups and therapists.

OCD-UK
P.O. Box 8955
Nottingham NG10, 9AU, United Kingdom
Website: www.ocduk.org

OCD-UK is similar to OCD Action and provides information on BDD, links to support groups, a listing of research studies, and other resources.

InfraPsych Australia
Website: www.infrapsych.com/root/1033/general/general_bdd.htm

InfraPsych Australia is a health company focused on developing services that improve clinical outcomes and reduce suffering. Its BDD site (designed by Roberta Honigman and Professor David J. Castle, who is an internationally recognized BDD expert) offers information to patients and health professionals about the symptoms of BDD and related disorders. It also offers some guidance for family members, as well as suggestions for further reading.

National Alliance on Mental Illness
Colonial Place Three
2107 Wilson Boulevard, Suite 300
Arlington, VA 22201-3042
Phone: 800-950-NAMI (6264)
Website: www.nami.org

The National Alliance on Mental Illness (NAMI) is a nonprofit, self-help, support and advocacy organization of patients, families, and friends of people with severe mental illnesses. NAMI provides education and support, helps with referrals, combats stigma, and supports increased funding for research.

Mental Health America
2000 North Beauregard Street, 6th floor
Alexandria, VA 22311
Phone: 800-969-6MHA (6642); 703-684-7722
Website: www.nmha.org

Mental Health America is dedicated to improving mental health and to preventing mental disorders through advocacy, education, and research.

Books

It is also a good idea to educate yourself about your BDD by reading the current literature related to this disorder. Therefore, in addition to reading this book, it may be helpful to check out the following books:

The Broken Mirror: Understanding and Treating Body Dysmorphic Disorder by Dr. Katharine A. Phillips (Oxford University Press, revised and expanded 2005). This comprehensive, groundbreaking volume complements this book, because it provides very detailed information on both the symptoms and pharmacotherapy treatment for BDD. It is helpful reading for people with BDD, their families, and clinicians.

The Adonis Complex: How to Identify, Treat, and Prevent Body Obsessions in Men and Boys by Harrison G. Pope, Jr., Katharine A. Phillips, and Roberto Olivardia (Free Press, 2000). This book, written for a male readership, provides useful information on muscle dysmorphia, BDD, and eating disorders.

Exacting Beauty: Theory, Assessment and Treatment of Body Image Disturbance by J.

Kevin Thompson, Leslie J. Heinberg, Madeline Altabe, and Stacy Tantleff-Dunn (American Psychological Association, 1999). This book provides a scholarly review of the research on body image and might help you better understand the complexities of your body image dissatisfaction.

The Body Myth: Adult Women and the Pressure to Be Perfect by Margo Maine and Joe Kelly (Wiley, 2005). This book was written for women with eating disorders and weight and shape concerns. Nevertheless, the chapter on culture and the media in particular might help you explore the forces that lead to body image dissatisfaction. The book also has many good strategies for dealing with negative attitudes related to aging.

Everything You Need to Know about Body Dysmorphic Disorder: Dealing with a Distorted Body Image by Pamela Walker (Rosen, 1999). This book, part of a series called Need to Know Library, is for children in grades 6 and up. It provides useful information for children and adolescents with BDD.

Focus on Body Image: How You Feel about How You Look by Maurene J. Hinds (Enslow, 2002). This book addresses how teens feel about their appearance and the impact of society and the media on body image. In addition to BDD and muscle dysmorphia, anorexia nervosa, binge-eating disorder, and bulimia nervosa are all briefly covered, and lists of their warning signs, as well as information on prevention and treatment, are included.

When Perfect Isn't Good Enough: Strategies for Coping with Perfectionism by Martin M. Anthony and Richard Swinson (New Harbinger, 1998). This book contains many practical strategies for anyone who struggles with excessive perfectionism (as so many people with body image problems do).

Journal Articles

In addition to reading books, you might want to check out PubMed on the Internet, a service of the National Library of Medicine that includes over 15 million citations for professional articles in life science journals. PubMed can be found at www.ncbi.nlm.nih.gov/entrez/query.fcgi. Just enter the topic of interest (for example, body dysmorphic disorder) as a search term to view a listing of relevant articles.

Index

About the Author

Sabine Wilhelm, PhD, is the founder and director of the Body Dysmorphic Disorder (BDD) Clinic and Research Unit at Massachusetts General Hospital and Associate Professor at Harvard Medical School, Boston, Massachusetts. She is internationally recognized as a leading researcher in BDD and is the principal investigator of two studies investigating treatments for the disorder funded by the National Institute of Mental Health. Her areas of clinical and research interest include the diagnosis and treatment of BDD, obsessive–compulsive disorder, and Tourette's disorder. She lives with her family near Boston.